Social and Emotional Development in Children through Emerging Adults

This concise guide offers an introduction to how children and young people develop social and emotional competence, and how they display appropriate social behavior and emotional expression at different ages.

Explaining the role of adults in a range of contexts and settings, this volume offers strategies for supporting competence and highlights key topics, such as attachment, prosocial behavior, social perspective taking, ethnic identity, social and emotional learning, gender identity, parenting styles, and much more. Moving through the different ages of childhood to emerging adulthood, the authors detail social and emotional development and the development of the self. They also offer strategies to foster social–emotional competence through these different ages.

Social and Emotional Development in Children through Emerging Adults is designed for students and professionals in psychological, educational, health and social work settings who want to support and nurture children and young people to ensure their needs are met.

Christi Crosby Bergin has worked as a professor and researcher in child and adolescent development for over 30 years. Currently, she is Director of the Prosocial Development and Education Research Lab at the University of Missouri. The lab is a group of faculty, postdoctoral fellows, and graduate students who study how to promote social–emotional competencies in children and youth. She earned a BS in psychology from Brigham Young University, and both an EdS and PhD from Stanford University.

Kimberly A. Gordon Biddle has a PhD from Stanford University in child and adolescent development. She is an American Psychological Association MFP fellow. She has been a college professor for 28 years. This is her third co-authored textbook. She is the author or co-author of over 15 peer-reviewed articles and some book chapters, a presenter or co-presenter of more than 35 peer-reviewed presentations, and the winner of one of the Stanford GSE Alumni Awards for Excellence in Education for 2018.

Applying Child and Adolescent Development in the Professions Series

Kimberly A. Gordon Biddle, *Emeritus Professor of Child and Adolescent Development, Sacramento State, California, USA*

The field of Child and Adolescent Development is being recognized and legitimized more and more as good preparation for a variety of careers in various fields such as; psychology, education, allied health, non-profits, and social work. As more theories are created and research is conducted, more attention and recognition is given to the field of Child and Adolescent Development.

This series will take core and current topics in the field of Child and Adolescent Development, define these topics, describe these topics as they develop in children from infancy to age 25 or describe how the topic impacts children from infancy to age 25, and then apply them to careers in five main fields: psychology, education, allied health, non-profits, and social work. Various application strategies and techniques will be shared. The core topics addressed in this series of books are as follows: attachment, motivation, social and emotional competence, executive function, and multilingual and multicultural development. The current niche topics represented in the series are these: transformative frames for anti-racism, socio-cultural deprivation, and growth mindset for transformative thinking. The writing level is to be accessible and engaging for students in high school and the first or second year of college. However, the information may be useful for graduate students, too. These books are excellent for early, mid, and late career professionals as well. Employee training and professional development can be enriched with the books of this series.

It is the intention of the book authors that our books are helpful to all people who work with and care for children. Indeed, the 8 books of the Applying Child and Adolescent Development in the Professions Series move the field forward.

Dr. Kimberly A. Gordon Biddle spent over 30 years working full-time in the field of Child and Adolescent Development, with 2 years as a Research Analyst and 28 plus years as a College Professor. Currently, she is an Emeritus Professor of Child and Adolescent Development from Sacramento State in California. Her BA is in Psychology and Music from the University of Redlands. Her EdS is in Program Evaluation and her PhD is in Child and Adolescent Development. Both of her advanced degrees are from Stanford University.

Over her career she has been an American Psychological Association MFP fellow. She has authored or co-authored over 20 articles and some book chapters. She has presented or co-presented over 40 presentations. Before being the overall editor of this series she had co-authored or co-edited 3 textbooks. This is her fourth textbook and it is co-authored with Dr. Christi Crosby Bergin. She has obtained approximately $1,000,000 in grants. Her research and teaching areas of expertise include motivation, academic resilience, social and emotional development, and the education and socialization of marginalized groups. She also has some expertise in field work placement and coordination and policies concerning children and families. Her career efforts have been rewarded. For example, she has received Outstanding Teaching and Service Awards from Sacramento State. She also won a Stanford Graduate School of Education Award for Excellence in Education in 2018 and a Career Award from the University of Redlands in 2019.

She is thrilled that Editor Helen Pritt at Routledge asked her to be the lead editor of this book series and she has enjoyed nurturing the series into life. She is happy to now be working with editor Molly Selby. This series is near and dear to her heart and she is honored to edit it and co-author one of the books. She firmly believes that this book series will move the field of Child and Adolescent Development forward. Core concepts of the field and current topics of the field are explored and applied in an engaging manner. Dr. Biddle firmly believes that knowledge of the field of Child and Adolescent Development can assist so many people, whether they are family members of children or are in careers working with children. This series aims to assist those in a wide range of careers who work with children. Those aims are met and surpassed in this series in the opinion of Dr. Biddle. It is her hope that this series is used with students in secondary, undergraduate, and graduate education settings in addition to adults in the fields of education, psychology, social work, allied health, and non-profit organizations. This series is the jewel in Dr. Biddle's career crown. She hopes it shines brightly.

From Cultural Deprivation to Cultural Security
Tackling Socio-Cultural Deprivation with Children and Young People
Dale Allender and Arya Allender-West

Social and Emotional Competence
A Short Guide for Professionals
Christi Crosby Bergin and Kimberly A. Gordon Biddle

For more information about this series, please visit: www.routledge.com/Applying-Child-and-Adolescent-Development-in-the-Professions-Series/book-series/ACADP

Social and Emotional Development in Children through Emerging Adults

A Guide for Professionals

Christi Crosby Bergin and
Kimberly A. Gordon Biddle

Routledge
Taylor & Francis Group

NEW YORK AND LONDON

Designed cover image: FatCamera via Getty Images

First published 2025
by Routledge
605 Third Avenue, New York, NY 10158

and by Routledge
4 Park Square, Milton Park, Abingdon, Oxon, OX14 4RN

Routledge is an imprint of the Taylor & Francis Group, an informa business

ISBN: 9780367495275 (hbk)
ISBN: 9780367495251 (pbk)
ISBN: 9781003046455 (ebk)

DOI: 10.4324/9781003046455

Typeset in Times New Roman
by Newgen Publishing UK

Contents

About the Authors

Christi Crosby Bergin has worked as a professor and researcher in child and adolescent development for over 30 years. Currently, she is the Director of the Prosocial Development and Education Research Lab at the University of Missouri. The lab is a group of faculty, postdoctoral fellows, and graduate students who study how to promote social–emotional competencies in children and youth. She earned a BS in psychology from Brigham Young University, and both an EdS and PhD from Stanford University.

She is a national expert in social–emotional development, with emphasis on prosocial behavior. She serves as the Chair of the Social and Emotional Learning Special Interest Group for the American Educational Research Association. She has served as Associate Dean of Research and Innovation in the College of Education and Human Development at MU. She was director of research at a medical center for programs designed to promote healthy development of prenatally drug-exposed children. She is a member of the Society for Research in Child Development, the European Association for Research on Learning and Instruction, and the Relation Centered Education Network. She has received teaching awards, paper and book awards, and an innovation award for creating the Network for Education Effectiveness that has hundreds of school district members. She was an owner of a small research business for several years. She has obtained over $60 million in competitive research grants from the U.S. Department of Education, the Centers for Disease Control, and the Department of Health and Human Services. She has 30 publications in peer-reviewed research journals, a textbook on child development in its fourth edition, with an international edition, a book for teachers, nine book chapters, and over 80 presentations at research conferences.

She is passionate about promoting children's well-being in all settings. Her work has straddled medical centers, schools, and therapeutic settings. She has consulted with educators, mental health providers, school boards, state and federal leaders and legislators on promoting prosocial behavior in children and adolescents. She is committed to taking research into practice, by helping professionals effectively use the research generated by scientists.

This book is intended to give you the knowledge and tools you need to promote the social–emotional well-being of every child whose life you touch for good. We hope you share our passion for helping children flourish.

Kimberly A. Gordon Biddle spent over 30 years working full-time in the field of child and adolescent development, with 2 years as a research analyst and 28 plus years as a college professor. Currently, she is Emeritus Professor of Child and Adolescent Development from Sacramento State in California. Her BA is in Psychology and Music from the University of Redlands. Her EdS is in Program Evaluation and her PhD is in Child and Adolescent Development. Both of her advanced degrees are from Stanford University.

Over her career, she has been an American Psychological Association MFP fellow. She has authored or co-authored over 20 articles and some book chapters. She has presented or co-presented over 40 presentations. Before being the overall editor of this series, she had co-authored or co-edited three textbooks. This is her fourth textbook and it is co-authored with Dr. Christi Crosby Bergin. She has obtained approximately $1,000,000 in grants. Her research and teaching areas of expertise include motivation, academic resilience, social and emotional development, and the education and socialization of marginalized groups. She also has some expertise in field work placement and coordination and policies concerning children and families. Her career efforts have been rewarded. For example, she has received Outstanding Teaching and Service Awards from Sacramento State. She also won Stanford Graduate School of Education Award for Excellence in Education in 2018 and Career Award from the University of Redlands in 2019.

She is thrilled that Editor Helen Pritt at Routledge asked her to be the lead editor of this book series and she has enjoyed nurturing the series into life. She is happy to now be working with editor Molly Selby. This series is near and dear to her heart and she is honored to edit it and co-author one of the books. She firmly believes that this book series will move the field of child and adolescent development forward. Core concepts of the field and current topics of the field are explored and applied in an engaging manner. Dr. Kimberly A. Gordon Biddle firmly believes that knowledge of the field of child and adolescent development can assist so many people, whether they are family members of children or are in careers working with children. This series aims to assist those in a wide range of careers who work with children. Those aims are met and surpassed in this series in the opinion of Dr. Kimberly Gordon Biddle. It is her hope that this series is used with students in secondary, undergraduate, and graduate education settings in addition to adults in the fields of education, psychology, social work, allied health, and non-profit organizations. This series is the jewel in Dr. Kimberly Gordon Biddle's career crown. She hopes it shines brightly.

Series Editor Foreword

The field of child and adolescent development is in infant stages of development, but it is steadily maturing. It is time for it be recognized and legitimized. As the theorizing and conduct of research in the field become more solid, complex, and applicable to life; recognition comes that the field is for people in a variety of professions. The traditional education and psychology fields are enriched with the knowledge obtained from the field of child and adolescent development. Additionally, allied health, social work, and non-profit fields are improved with knowledge of how to apply child and adolescent development research in the workplace. Everyone who works with or cares for children from birth to 25 years will benefit from reading and applying the information from the books in this series. Collectively, the authors have created books rich with foundational information and application techniques and strategies. Thematic boxes of interviews, case studies, and research and theory into practice run throughout all the books. These books help to answer some of the most important questions concerning children and their development. All who love and care about children should read every book in the series.

It is a definite highlight of my career to have co-authored this book with Dr. Christi Crosby Bergin. Her knowledge of social and emotional competence is unsurpassed. Her experience in textbook writing is noteworthy. Our textbook on social and emotional competence is a must read for everyone who works with children of all ages. Topics include attachment, prosocial behavior, social perspective taking, ethnic identity, social and emotional learning (SEL), gender identity, parenting styles, and much more. As with all books in this series, strategies for implementation are included. Readers will find methods for enriching social and emotional competence in all ages of children in this textbook. This book is necessary reading for all adults in all settings that interact with children from birth to age 25, from classrooms to therapeutic and medical settings. It is especially enlightening for parents and all child and adolescent professionals.

Acknowledgments

An abundance of thanks goes to Mr. Caison Del Valle for drawing ten figure images for this textbook with style and speed.

There are many people to thank for supporting us during the writing process. First, I want to thank my husband, Chris, and son, Emmanuel, for all of their cheerleading and support during this journey. I also thank my mom, Mary, and brother, Randy. The support of loved ones is invaluable. I also want to thank the CSU – Emeritus and Retired Faculty and Staff Association for their support through the Small Grants program. Thanking my Sacramento Country Day School interns for their research and administrative assistance is a must. So, a big thank you goes to Annabelle Do, Grace Zhao, Zoe Genetos, Milly Wong, Priya Chand, and Callister Misquitta. Certainly, I am thankful to God who makes all things possible.

- Kimberly A. Gordon Biddle

I thank Dr. Kimberly Gordon Biddle for asking me to co-write this book with her. I will miss our regular joint writing sessions and chats as we prepared this book. Special thanks goes to my husband, David Bergin, who uncomplainingly did the tedious work of editing our writing and brought food to my desk during writing marathons. I thank my children – all four of them, their spouses, and the 10 grandchildren they have brightened my life with – for constantly giving me material for my writing. I thank my sisters for long conversations about the challenges their patients and students face; they remind me of why my work, and yours, is important.

- Christi Crosby Bergin

Chapter 1

Emotional Competence

Imagine Rob is in your small group at school. He doesn't do his share of the work and seems constantly angry in class. You feel angry with Rob and are about to tell him off. Before you do, another student tells you: "His mother is seriously ill and lost her job three months ago. He's worried sick they might lose their home. He'll never tell you because he thinks 'worry' is for weaklings; it's so much easier to be angry." Your emotion changes to compassion instead of anger.

Just what are emotions like anger and compassion? Can you control them? How can you be more accurate in reading other's emotions, like Rob's worry? This chapter will help you answer these and other questions.

What Are Emotions and Why Do You Have Them?

You know what the word "emotion" means, but try to define it and you'll find it is not as straight forward as you might think. Here's how psychologists define it: An "emotion" is a subjective reaction to an important event that involves physiological change, readiness to act, and interpretation of the event (Gross, 2015). Let's unpack this definition. First, it is subjective, meaning it is unique to how you see a situation. Second, you have emotions in response to events that are important to you. If you do not care about an event, you are not likely to feel emotion about it. Third, emotions are characterized by changes in your body, like a racing heart rate, burning cheeks, and rising temperature. Fourth, these changes in your body make you ready to take action, like running away when you feel fear. Fifth, the emotions you feel depend on how you interpret an event. As you saw in the example of Rob above, *changes in the way you interpret an event lead to different emotions.* Remember this last point because reappraisal of events can make you and others happier. We will come back to this point.

Think about how these five components are different for two common emotions. You feel *anger* when you interpret an event as an attack on someone you care about; your face flushes, your eyes narrow, your heart races, and you are motivated to counterattack. You feel *shame* when you interpret an event as

DOI: 10.4324/9781003046455-1

having let others down through your mistake; your cheeks flush, you slump, your eyes are downcast, your heart slows, you smile weakly, and you are motivated to hide from others. These are just two examples. The next time you feel a strong emotion, notice how the five components of emotions work together.

Emotions are important. They help you have laser-like focus on important events, prepare for action, and motivate you to do something. Generally positive emotions, like interest, cause you to focus on and approach something. In contrast, negative emotions, like fear, cause you to focus on and avoid something. Emotions also help with communication. When your mother scowled at you for walking into the house with dirty shoes, you probably took them off quickly. Emotions also improve your thinking. When you feel positive emotions – like interest, happiness, or excitement – you tend to be more creative, productive, open to new information, and perform better on tasks. Even negative emotions, *if they are mild and temporary*, can help your thinking. For example, a little anxiety motivates you to better prepare for a presentation.

Although emotions serve important functions, they are not always beneficial. Any emotion can be a problem if it is out of control, whether it is momentary or long-term. For example, if you experience chronic shame, you might become aggressive and develop low self-esteem. For another example, if you feel very angry right now, you will have a hard time focusing on reading this chapter because strong negative emotions swamp your thoughts.

Given that negative emotions can swamp our thinking, we may not remember, learn, or make good decisions when experiencing *intense* negative emotions. Imagine a teacher mocks a student who gets a math problem wrong and then tells how to do the problem correctly. The shame and embarrassment that flood the student's thoughts make it unlikely the student will remember the correct procedure. This is why intense embarrassment, anxiety, or sadness can make people seem less intelligent. Thus, *helping children learn to better regulate their emotions may be more important to their success than helping them develop greater knowledge or skills.*

What Is Emotional Competence?

Children who are emotionally competent have two key abilities: (1) the ability to regulate their own emotions and (2) the ability to understand others' emotions. Let's discuss each (see Figure 1.1).

Emotion Regulation: What It Is and Why It Matters

Emotion regulation is the ability to change the intensity and duration of your emotions to fit the situation (Gross, 2015). For example, you might be angry at your boss, but you need to dampen that anger in order to keep your job. Alternatively, if you feel someone has been wronged, you might need to stoke

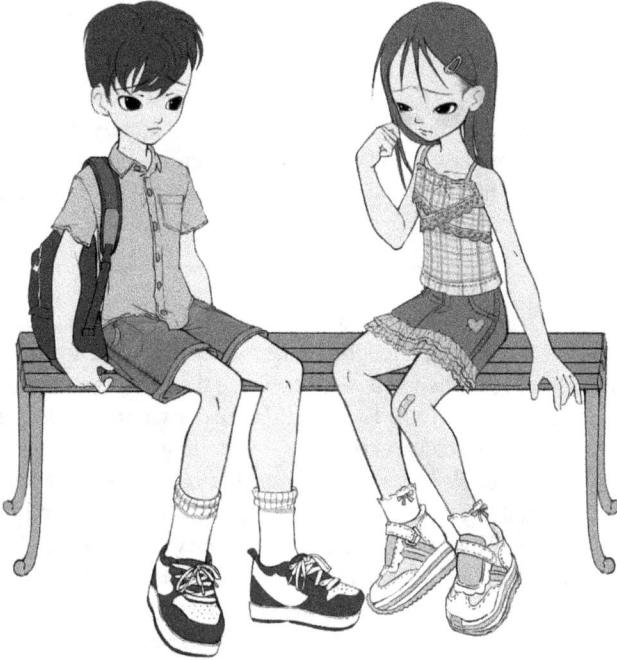

Figure 1.1 Emotional competence includes the ability to regulate your own emotions and read other's emotions accurately.

your anger so that you can stand up to the wrong doer. How do you regulate your emotions? You use coping strategies, which are listed in Box 1.1.

Coping strategies refer to your deliberate attempt to change your emotions when you feel overwhelmed by emotion. Coping strategies can be either: (1) *problem-focused* or (2) *emotion-focused.* Problem-focused coping strategies are attempts to change the situation or solve the problem. For example, if you feel shame over letting your team down on a group assignment, you work harder. Emotion-focused coping strategies are attempts to change your emotions, such as changing the way you think about the situation or seeking comfort from others. For example, if you feel shame over letting your team down on a group assignment, you may attempt to reduce your shame by talking with your friends about how useless the assignment was or how other members of the group did not do their fair share.

Box 1.1 Coping Strategies

<u>Less Constructive Strategies</u>: Do nothing. Aggress (snatch, hit, kick, throw things). Use drugs or alcohol. Cry. Withdraw. Ruminate (rehash and dwell on it over and over).

<u>More Constructive Strategies</u>: Take action to fix the situation. Reappraise (think about the situation in a positive way or change your goal). Pray or meditate. Talk with wise others. Fake it. Exercise or relax (depending on whether it is a high-arousal or low-arousal emotion). Seek help from others. Distract yourself.

Which coping strategy should you use? That depends on the situation. When you have some control over the situation, problem-focused strategies may be more helpful. However, when you cannot change the situation, emotion-focused strategies may be more helpful. Even within these two broad categories, some approaches may be less constructive (e.g., punching the wall, getting drunk) than other approaches. *Reappraisal is often the best strategy* when you cannot change the situation. In the example about Rob above, the other student's explanation of his family situation can cause you to *reappraise* Rob's behavior and change your emotions toward him; you feel more empathy and less anger. Reappraisal is effective and does not wear down your self-control as much as some other strategies. It is a great tool to use in a variety of situations.

Another effective strategy is to "fake it." When you express no emotion or an emotion that is different (but more acceptable) from what you actually feel, you are using *emotional dissemblance*. Some people mistakenly believe that if you keep emotions locked up, they might explode. This volcano myth is false. Emotions fade if they are not expressed. In addition, when you fake being happy even though you are not, you tend to feel happier. Think about a time you didn't want to go to a party because you felt gloomy, but you went and smiled at everyone. You probably left the party feeling happier. There may be a physical explanation for this. As you smile, your facial muscles provide feedback to the brain, which then alters your emotion.

Emotional dissemblance is an important skill because it helps you fit in with your culture. Cultures have rules about what emotions can be expressed when and to whom. For example, a 10-year-old expressing anger toward grandma for giving a lame birthday gift is not considered acceptable in most cultures. You can probably think of many examples from your own culture about emotions that you should or should not display toward teachers, police officers, and coaches. Emotional dissemblance helps you become successful in your culture.

Even very young children can dissemble, although it is a sophisticated skill to know the rules for what emotion to display, understand how others will react to their emotions, and control their emotional display. Like many skills, emotional dissemblance can be used for good or ill. When children use it to protect others' feelings (e.g., grandma who gave an undesirable gift), it is generally good. When children use emotional dissemblance to lie or harm others, it is not good.

Reading Others' Emotions: What It Is and Why It Matters

Thus far, we have discussed the important skill of regulating your own emotions. The second crucial part of emotional competence is being able to read others' emotions accurately. This skill is called *affective perspective-taking*. (*Affective* means related to mood, feelings, and emotions.) Affective perspective-taking is essential for success in your social world. For example, imagine you are in a meeting with someone whose brow is furrowed. You need to be able to discern whether the person is angry or just concentrating hard so that you can respond appropriately.

When affective perspective-taking involves sharing feelings with another person in distress, we call it *empathy*. Empathy can cause you to respond in three ways: (1) You can feel *sympathy*, which is feeling concern for the other's feelings. This leads you to help the person in distress. (2) You can feel *personal distress*, which is focused on your own discomfort. This might lead you to help the other, but it is more likely to lead you to avoid the situation. (3) You can feel *empathic distress*, which is feeling along with the other person. This leads you to help the other person and promotes deeper relationships.

Your ability to read others' emotions not only helps you feel with others, but it also helps you understand ambiguous situations. For example, imagine in a meeting someone announces that you have been assigned 30 patient cases to manage. You do not know whether this is a typical or an outrageous number, so you look at the reactions of others in the room. Open mouths and raised eyebrows suggest it is outrageous. This is called *social referencing* because you are referencing others' reactions for information about a situation that is ambiguous to you. Try to notice the next time you use it.

One way you can feel *with* others is through *emotion contagion*. This means the emotions of one person trigger similar emotions in another. For example, if you hear a joke that is not very funny, but another person is laughing heartily, you might laugh too. Humans are hardwired to catch the emotions of others. Emotion contagion is unintentional, and it can actually change your emotions. Emotion contagion is a wonderful asset because it helps you relate to other people and experience empathy, but it can also result in false memories (e.g., believing you experienced something that actually you only saw someone else experience), and it can result in personal distress, rather than sympathy, which might lead you to turn away from a person in distress.

How Does Emotional Competence Change with Age?

Overall, your ability to regulate your emotions should have improved dramatically since birth. Newborns have a few very rudimentary strategies for coping with strong emotions. For example, they may look away, suck their hand, or appear to sleep. They need adult support to regulate their emotions. Toddlers have some emotion regulation ability; for example, they can often refrain from crying when they fall down, but when they get an adult's attention, their restraint is overcome and they howl with gusto. However, toddlers continue to need support from adults (e.g., rocking, cuddling) to soothe big emotions. Box 1.2 illustrates how you can help toddlers learn to regulate their emotions. This case study comes from an interview with Kathy, a preschool teacher.

Box 1.2   Preschool Case Study

I often help children calm down and get to their original emotional state by holding them in my lap and just rocking them until the children are able to take deep breaths with me and they are able to calm down. Then, I ask them what happened and why they are so upset. If the children are verbal, they answer me. If not, I try to discern what happened and talk to them to help them regulate their emotions more.

Preschoolers are able to regulate their own emotions under normal conditions, although they are better at exaggerating than at squelching an emotion. They practice regulating emotions through pretend play, so you may see them "trying on" different emotions as they play, such as angrily spanking a naughty doll but then kissing and hugging it, or angrily fighting a foe as they pretend to be superheroes. Coping skills continue to improve incrementally until by age 10 most children have almost adult-like ability to regulate their emotions. By this age, children have more coping strategies in their toolbox and are able to better judge which strategy would be most helpful in a situation. They can control their emotions enough to fake out onlookers (e.g., pretending they like a gift that they do not really like).

In contrast, ability to read others' emotions may develop faster than emotion regulation. This is because empathy, emotion contagion, and social referencing are already present in infants. Within the first days of life, infants can mimic others' facial expressions and can tell one emotion from another. Within a few months, they will also be able to use social referencing to tell whether something is safe (e.g., reading their parents' emotional expressions to know whether it is safe to let another adult hold them).

Although it is present in infants, the ability to read others' emotions grows in the preschool years as children learn to label and talk about emotions (e.g., my sister is *angry* because I took her ball). We know that preschoolers even understand the causes of others' emotions because they will deliberately tease siblings to get an emotional reaction (e.g., stand in front of the TV when a sibling is watching a show) or comfort others in distress (e.g., bring a comfort blanket to a sibling who is crying).

By middle childhood, children can understand that someone might have multiple, competing emotions in the same situation, and they become more accurate in discussing and labeling others' emotions. By adolescence, as teens' cognitive skills develop, they can become empathic to people in faraway countries. At the same time, they can also become more self-protective so that generally, they *are not more empathic toward others* compared to their younger selves. For example, if a boy trips and falls in front of others, they may be less likely to say "That happened to me also" and help him up, compared to younger children. Through adulthood, people continue to grow in their ability to read others' emotions. We'll discuss the emotional milestones and skills associated with different ages in greater detail in Chapters 3–6.

In What Ways Do Individuals Differ in Emotional Competence?

While there are clear general age trends in the development of emotional competence, two children of the same age can differ in their level of emotional competence.

Typical Variation

Children differ in how quickly they feel emotions, how intense their emotions are, and how quickly they recover equilibrium. Some feel chronic negative emotions. Some feel too little emotion; for example, children who experience abuse may develop blunted emotions.

How do these differences affect children? Emotional competence is an important asset. Those who are good at emotion regulation are better liked by others around them. They more often feel positive, rather than negative, emotions, which leads to less aggression and more positive behavior, smoother social interactions, and better friendships. When children are happy, they greet others more warmly, engage with them, and make activities pleasant so that people want to be around them.

Children who are good at *emotion regulation* also tend to have better language skills and higher grades and test scores because: (1) they are liked better by teachers and classmates and (2) they can keep emotions from swamping their ability to pay attention and learn in school. In fact, school-based interventions that reduce K-12 students' emotional distress also indirectly raise their grades and test scores. In contrast, children with poor emotion regulation are at risk for being disliked by others if they are often angry. Anger makes others uncomfortable, and angry children may be aggressive or act out at school which can short-circuit their learning opportunities.

Similarly, children with better *affective perspective-taking* skills and more empathy than others of their age are liked and sought out by peers. Perhaps this is because they are also less aggressive, less annoying, more cooperative, and better able to establish rapport with others (Tan et al., 2022). They also have greater self-control and higher achievement at school (Voltmer & von Salisch, 2017). In contrast, children with low ability to read other's emotions are less liked by peers and tend to be aggressive. They often misinterpret emotion cues, such as mistaking sad expressions for anger.

These two aspects of emotional competence – regulating one's own emotions and reading others' emotions – influence each other. You need to accurately read others' emotions (e.g., "he's sad") to select the most appropriate coping strategy (e.g., "help him reappraise"), and then monitor others' responses to decide whether to change your strategy (e.g., "he just wanted a hug"). You have to regulate your own emotions in order to respond sympathetically rather than with personal distress.

Biological Basis of Differences in Emotional Competence

Perhaps there is a small biological basis to differences in emotional competence. Some children are born with a bent toward negative emotions that appears in the first months of life and remains somewhat stable. Thus, irritable children are not likely to just outgrow their negativity unless their social environment is supportive. Furthermore, there is some evidence that depression and anxiety may share a small underlying genetic predisposition (Rhee et al., 2015). However, keep in mind that genes alone do not cause emotional disorders. Rather, they make some children *more vulnerable to the effects of their social environment*, such as negative parenting or life stress. For example, research suggests that young children with genetic predisposition toward negative emotions may become more negative than the average child if they have depressed, unresponsive, or unhappily married parents. However, the same predisposition may cause them to be *more happy* than the average child if their parents are happy (Dadds et al., 2015).

Social Basis of Differences in Emotional Competence

Research robustly finds that children's emotional competence is strongly influenced by experience, especially experience with their parents. Children with good emotion regulation and good affective perspective-taking skills have parents who accept their emotional displays without over-reacting, express positive emotions at home, talk about emotions during sibling conflict, and are supportive. They have parents who communicate that they enjoy their children. Perhaps most importantly, children with good emotion regulation have secure attachment to their parents. Attachment is discussed in Chapter 2. Young securely attached children whose parents are sensitive tend to grow into adolescents who have good coping strategies, are able to take on emotionally charged situations constructively, and are less likely to become depressed. In contrast, children who have anxious, insecure attachment to their parents are more likely to experience personal distress in emotionally charged situations rather than sympathy. As adolescents, they find it more difficult to control their emotions in constructive ways. We will discuss how parents establish secure attachment in Chapter 2.

Children's developing brains adapt to their social environments. This can be a good thing, but it also can make children living in toxic environments vulnerable to stress. A little stress is okay, and most children will cope just fine. But chronic and high levels of stress can impair the brain's ability to regulate emotions. This is why chronic stress leaves children vulnerable to emotional disorders. They are more affected by daily stress than other children and less able to regulate their emotions.

Emotional Disorders

Some children are very poor at regulating their emotions. This condition is called an *emotional disorder*. Emotional disorders can be either externalizing or internalizing. *Externalizing disorders* involve aggression, anger, and acting out. *Internalizing disorders* involve withdrawal or sadness. The two most common disorders in childhood are depression and anxiety, which are both internalizing disorders, and they tend to occur together. A child can have *both* internalizing and externalizing disorders, such as being depressed, anxious, and aggressive. Almost half (40%) of children with one disorder have another disorder as well.

Emotional disorders are common and becoming more common. Prior to the COVID-19 pandemic, about 22% of all children, or one in four or five, had at least one serious disorder before reaching adulthood (Avenevoli et al., 2015). During the decade leading to the pandemic (2009–2019) the proportion of high-school students reporting persistent sadness or hopelessness increased by 40% (CDC, 2020). To make matters worse, there was a rapid global rise of emotional disorders during the pandemic (SAMSHA, 2022).

What do these disorders look like? Children with *internalizing disorders* worry more and feel sad or angry more than other children. They have difficulty using a variety of coping strategies, so they find it more challenging to

Table 1.1 Symptoms of Common Emotional Disorders in Children

Internalizing disorders		Externalizing disorder
Depression	Anxiety	Conduct disorder
Median age of onset 11 (mild)/13 (major)	Median age of onset 6 years	Median age of onset 8–15 years[a]
Irritability	Irritability	Irritability
Social withdrawal	Poor concentration	Aggressive
Poor concentration	Can't-sit-still behavior	Consistently violate
Lack of interest in school	(e.g., foot kicking, hair twirling, mouth	social norms and the rights of others
Feeling worthless	touching, lip licking,	Little guilt or empathy
Changes in appetite	lip twisting, crying,	Assume others are acting
Self-criticism	chewing on objects,	with hostile intent
Poor hygiene	and nail biting)	toward them
Can't-sit-still behavior		Hyperactivity,
Frequent crying		inattention, and
Sleep problems		impulsivity

Source: American Psychiatric Association (2022).

Notes:
[a] Childhood vs. adolescent onset have different diagnoses; in early to middle childhood similar behaviors may present as oppositional defiant disorder.
Anxiety is different from fear. Fear is an emotional response to an immediate threat to safety. Anxiety is a feeling of helplessness focused on future threats or on threats to the sense of self.

recruit positive emotions and squelch negative emotions. Children with conduct disorder (CD), an *externalizing disorder*, are chronically and excessively disruptive or aggressive. Classic symptoms of common disorders are listed in Table 1.1. Any child might have these symptoms occasionally. For example, children may cling and have sleep problems when they move to a new house. However, if symptoms are severe for at least 2 weeks, or less severe but last for several months or more, they may indicate an emotional disorder. Treatment is more effective if it begins early, yet most children with emotional disorders do not get help developing better emotion regulation.

Emotion regulation disorders can be manifest at any age. Anxiety is apparent in some toddlers, and you may see some toddlers diagnosed with depression. However, the median age for onset of diagnosable anxiety disorders is age 6 (meaning that half are diagnosed younger and half are diagnosed older). The median age for onset of mild depression is age 11 and major depression is age 13. Rates of depression rise during adolescence, peak around ages 15–17, and then decrease. CD is typically manifest between middle childhood and middle adolescence.

Emotional disorders are significant risk factors for children. Being frequently anxious, unhappy, or angry is distressing enough. But in addition, children with emotional disorders often have other co-morbidities (i.e., conditions that go together), including Attention Deficit Hyperactivity Disorder (ADHD), learning disorders, and eating disorders (Rhee et al., 2015). They tend to have more illnesses, school absences, dropping out, poor grades, low test scores (for their IQ), drug abuse, recklessness, and injury proneness than other children. In addition, they tend to be lonely because peers do not want to play with them. Children who learn good coping strategies, rather than destructive or escapist strategies, are likely to recover. This is why early intervention is important.

Insecure attachment to parents, discussed in Chapter 2, may be the primary underlying cause of emotional disorders. Other risk factors include marital conflict, domestic violence, parenting style (see Chapter 4), parents who use harsh discipline or are hypercritical, and negative life events (e.g., death or divorce in the family). Parents who are anxious or depressed may pass on anxiety or depression through emotion contagion and compromised quality of parenting. Interview Box 1.3 illustrates how Leslie, a social worker, helps children with emotional disorders.

The more risk factors operating in a child's life, the more likely that child will experience one or more emotional disorders. Also, children who struggle with both internalizing and externalizing disorders are two to three times as likely to develop mental illness in adulthood compared to typical children.

Abuse

Abuse affects children's emotional competence. Abused children tend to either under- or over-regulate their emotions. Under-regulated children may feel overwhelming anger, fear, and shame. They may be volatile, rapidly shifting into these negative emotions because they are already swamped by emotion. Over-regulated abused children appear unfeeling. They have blunted emotions, blank or sober expressions, and are unresponsive to emotional events. They may refuse to talk about emotions or about the abuse. They suppress emotions because it helps them cope when they cannot escape the abuser or find protection. On the surface, this might appear adaptive, but unfortunately this rigid over-regulation prevents them from developing other coping skills. When their refusal to feel suddenly fails, they can be explosive because they do not have coping skills. Some may claim that the abuse was "no big deal" and that they are not affected by it, but then "cope" in destructive ways such as drug abuse, abusive friendships, and a variety of problem behaviors. Thus, a key treatment for abused children is to help them learn to communicate emotions and develop coping strategies.

Abused children also have difficulty reading others' emotions accurately. They are biased toward perceiving negative emotions in others like sadness and anger. This may be adaptive in the short-term because they need to watch for cues that an abusive event is imminent. However, in the long-term, this bias interferes with building healthy relationships. Their careful watchfulness of others' negativity can also consume their thinking capacity, making it more difficult to learn at school. Abuse also interferes with children's empathy. Abused children are more likely to respond to others' distress with their own distress and withdraw from those in need, rather than with sympathy. Or, they may attack and laugh at a peer who is in distress, because this is what has happened to them. They need support to learn how to watch, help, or comfort others in distress.

Box 1.3   Interview with a Social Worker

The following interview is with Leslie, a Licensed Clinical Social Worker.

What is your job?

I'm a group therapist for preteens (ages 11–13) with behavior issues from all over the county. They come to our facility after school for a couple hours each day. Kids get referred to us by administrators and teachers at school for having behavior issues. Or, a parent expresses concern about their child to a school counselor, who refers them to our program. They are low-income, and Medicaid pays for it. Their issues range widely from violent and threatening to depressed and suicidal. They must have some kind of diagnosis to be in our program such as ADHD, oppositional defiance disorder, CD, post-traumatic stress disorder (PTSD), depression, anxiety.

Each day we have a focus, such as anger management, friendship quality, or communication. We teach skills to the kids through discussion and activities. Most have ADHD-like behaviors and are sleep deprived. They are tired of school for the day, so we keep the "lesson" part to a minimum.

What role does emotional competence play in the needs of the kids?

Its HUGE! They don't have age-appropriate emotion regulation. They get sent to us because they just lose their mind – screaming obscenities and threatening the teacher or other students – whenever a teacher reprimands them. They mostly have externalizing disorders, but a small percentage of the kids are sent to us for depression.

Can you give me concrete examples that indicate poor emotion regulation?

I can give you plenty of examples because poor emotion regulation is core to their challenges. One example is that we use a reward system where the kids get a piece of candy for good behavior. If they don't earn a piece of candy, some kids throw things, rip things off the wall, or have a tantrum.

In another example, a girl has severe depression. For her, every little thing becomes a big, big emotional event. For example, some kids started a game of tag, but no one specifically asked her if she wanted to play tag. She stormed away and pouted until someone came and cajoled her into playing.

Another girl accidentally hit her friend with a ball during a game. The friend lost it. He screamed obscenities at her. The staff intervened, telling him that it was an accident and that the girl had apologized. He then turned on the staff, threatening to stab a staff member, throwing a chair, and trying to punch the staff. Staff had to hide the girl to protect her from her "friend."

Another girl picked up a pen from the ground thinking it was hers, but a boy claimed it. The boy is known as a chronic liar who steals, so no one believed him. He had tried to steal scissors a few days before and had stolen multiple fidget toys from the room. Others said it was the girls' pen. The boy stormed off, crying over a pen. The girl gave it to him. It still took him over an hour to calm down enough to come back to the room.

Another boy came to us with no emotion regulation ability. We have the kids do short, easy worksheets at times. Other times, we do a craft or color a picture. This boy, if he made a mistake or didn't understand something, would yell, storm off, or throw his head down on the table. After a year and a half in our program, he "graduated." He was doing much, much better, although his emotion regulation still wasn't completely age-appropriate. He quit storming out of the room and rarely yelled. He still sometimes put his head down, but started to use it more as a calming technique and would get back to the worksheet or ask for help after a few minutes.

What do you think causes these emotional disorders among your kids?

Our kids have high rates of parent loss and family dysfunction. Some moms "give them away" to grandparents because they prioritize a boyfriend over the kids. Probably, half live with a grandparent. When children's protective services are involved, they usually place them in kinship care, but some are in foster care. Some are adopted, but then the adoptive parents divorce, so they experience double abandonment. Others live with a single mom who can't manage them.

Most of the kids' guardians do not have good emotion regulation themselves. The kids are often hit or yelled at for infractions at home or if the school reported misbehavior to their guardians. So, the kids learn that yelling and fists should be used for emotional expression. The guardians also are typically authoritarian. If the kids try to excuse or explain their behavior, guardians interpret it as "talking back" or being "disrespectful." Sometimes guardians punish the kids by taking their game system or phone away. The kids aren't learning self-control or empathy at home.

I've noticed that the boys in our program often listen to the male staff more than the female staff. Gender and race make a difference. The kids listen more to staff who they identify with.

You've talked about their emotion regulation skills. What about their affective perspective-taking skills?

Most are OK, but some have problems reading others' emotions. Like they can't read that others are bored by a long story they are telling, or when others make snide remarks it goes over their heads. But, some are good at spotting when other people are angry or upset. Almost too good.

They tend toward low empathy, but are not completely unfeeling. If someone is upset, they will check in with each other and say "Hey, are you OK?"

Any concluding thoughts?

Emotion regulation can be learned. Some kids make improvements in our program. Their emotion regulation gets better, so they no longer stomp off or yell at others whenever something happens. As they get better at regulating their emotions, they also start having friends, which in turn improves their emotion regulation in a positive cycle.

In What Ways Do Groups Differ in Emotional Competence?

Research has found some differences in emotional competence based on gender, socio-economic status (SES) or poverty, and culture/ethnicity/race.

Gender

Girls tend to be better at emotion regulation compared to boys. As early as infancy, girls are less likely than boys to respond with anger if their mothers ignore them. In middle childhood, girls are better at faking being happy when they are not (i.e., emotional dissemblance). Girls tend to smile more than boys, which helps them control emotions and interact pleasantly (McDuff et al., 2017). Ironically, despite girls' advantage in emotion regulation, they also tend to have higher rates of anxiety and depression (US Surgeon General, 2021).

Research has not consistently found gender differences in *reading other's emotions*. Some studies find that girls are better at reading others' distress and showing concern for others, but some studies find no gender differences. Some researchers suggest that girls may have a slight push toward greater empathic distress which might explain girls' greater depression.

Socio-Economic Status (Poverty)

Research finds more consistent, but small, differences in emotion regulation based on SES than on gender. Children living in poverty tend to struggle with emotion regulation more than children who have more resources. They tend to have more stressors to cope with, those stressors cascade one after another, and children have fewer helpful adults to teach them coping skills. However, children living in poverty can develop good emotion regulation if adults help them in the ways discussed in later chapters.

Culture and Ethnicity

Culture refers to the customary beliefs, values, institutions, and behaviors of an ethnic/racial, religious, or social group. Your culture may be determined by where you live (continent, country, neighborhood), your race, ethnicity, religion, politics, SES, language, immigration status, or the era when you were born. Research finds that emotions are expressed similarly across cultures. That is, you can read others' emotions from cultures different from your own through facial expressions, tone of voice, and body language. However, there are subtle cultural differences, somewhat akin to different dialects of the same language. This means that you may be a little better at reading the emotions of members of your own culture.

There are some ethnic/racial differences in emotional disorders in the United States. Black youth are more likely to have anxiety disorders, and Latino youth are more likely to have depression, than White youth (Avenevoli et al., 2015). You might expect that immigrant youth would have more mental health issues because they must accommodate multiple cultures, sever relationships from their first country, struggle to speak the local language, and experience ethnic slurs. However, on average, they have similar or better mental health than non-immigrant peers (Morris et al., 2015). Among the minority of immigrant youth who do have emotional disorders, stress within the family is the primary risk factor, as it is for other youth.

Chapter Summary

Emotions serve important functions for your survival and well-being. They can help you focus, prepare for, and motivate you to take action, communicate with others, and improve your thinking. However, when they are out of control, they can lead to behavior problems and swamp your thinking. This is why emotional competence is defined as having two components: (1) Ability to regulate one's own emotions using constructive (rather than destructive) coping strategies. (2) Ability to read others' emotions accurately and feel empathy when appropriate. These abilities improve with age. Infants have minimal ability to regulate their emotions by themselves, but by age 10, adult-like emotion regulation ability is usually reached. Ability to read others' emotions is present in infancy through social contagion, yet the ability continues to grow into old age.

Individuals differ in emotional competence. Those with age-appropriate abilities are happier, better liked by others, and achieve more in school. Individual differences might have a biological basis, but they are primarily the result of social experience, particularly in the family. Stressful family environments may result in either internalizing or externalizing disorders. Fortunately, emotional competence can be improved; strategies are discussed in Chapters 3–11.

Suggested Readings

Barrett, L. (2018). *How emotions are made: The secret life of the brain.* Mariner.
Brackett, M. (2019). *Permission to feel: The power of emotional intelligence to achieve well-being and success.* Celadon/Macmillan.
DeSteno, D. (2018). *Emotional success: The motivational power of gratitude, compassion and pride.* Macmillan.
Gross, J. (2015). Emotion regulation: Current status and future prospects. *Psychological Inquiry, 26*(1), 1–26.

References

American Psychiatric Association. (2022). Diagnostic and statistical manual of mental disorders, 5th ed., text revision. Author.
Avenevoli, S., Swendsen, J., He, J.-P., Burstein, M., & Merikangas, K. (2015). Major depression in the National Comorbidity Survey-Adolescent Supplement: Prevalence, correlates, and treatment. *Journal of the American Academy of Child and Adolescent Psychiatry, 54*(1), 37–44.

Centers for Disease Control and Prevention. (2020). Youth Risk Behavior Survey Data Summary & Trends Report 2009–2019. Retrieved from www.cdc.gov/healthyyouth/data/yrbs/pdf/YRBSDataSummaryTrendsReport2019-508.pdf

Dadds, M. R., Moul, C., Hawes, D. J., Mendoza Diaz, A., & Brennan, J. (2015). Individual differences in childhood behavior disorders associated with epigenetic modulation of the cortisol receptor gene. *Child Development, 86*(5), 1311–1320.

Gross, J. (2015). Emotion regulation: Current status and future prospects. *Psychological Inquiry, 26*(1), 1–26.

McDuff, D., Kodra, E., Kaliouby, R. e., & LaFrance, M. (2017). A large-scale analysis of sex differences in facial expressions. *PLoS ONE, 12*(4), e0173942. https://doi.org/10.1371/journal.pone.0173942

Morris, M. W., Chiu, C.-y., & Liu, Z. (2015). Polycultural psychology. *Annual Review of Psychology, 66*(1), 631–659.

Rhee, S. H., Lahey, B. B., & Waldman, I. D. (2015). Comorbidity among dimensions of childhood psychopathology: Converging evidence from behavior genetics. *Child Development Perspectives, 9*(1), 26–31.

Substance Abuse and Mental Health Services Administration (SAMHSA). (2022). *National survey on drug use and health.*

Tan, L., Volling, B. L., Gonzalez, R., LaBounty, J., & Rosenberg, L. (2022). Growth in emotion understanding across early childhood: A cohort-sequential model of firstborn children across the transition to siblinghood. *Child Development, 93*(3), e299–e314.

US Surgeon General. (2021). *Protecting youth mental health.* Department of Health and Human Services.

Voltmer, K., & von Salisch, M. (2017). Three meta-analyses of children's emotion knowledge and their school success. *Learning and Individual Differences, 59*, 107–118.

Chapter 2

Social Competence

Jamal is a seventh grader who is well-liked by his classmates. When asked "who would you like to work with today?" the other students usually nominate Jamal. One day the students were working at the board together. An impulsive student, Amir, pushed his way in front of Jamal. Other students scolded, "Hey! Jamal was there first!" Amir looked a little worried about their scolding, which Jamal noticed. Jamal kindly patted Amir on the back and quietly said, "Its OK. You are doing fine. Go ahead."

Is Jamal's behavior typical for his age? Was Jamal kind toward Amir because he is compassionate? What can adults do to help children become kind like Jamal? This chapter will help you answer these and other questions.

In Chapter 1, you learned about emotional competence. In this chapter, you will learn about social competence. Emotional and social competence are strongly interrelated. In fact, they are often used in the same phrase, as in "social–emotional well-being." A person with strong emotional competence is likely to also have good social competence and vice versa. For example, understanding and accurately labeling your own and others' emotions (e.g., frustration, sadness, fear) helps you respond more constructively during social conflict (Collie, 2020). For another example, when you have healthy friendships, you tend to be happier. Notice at the end of the interview in Chapter 1, the social worker said that as the kids in her intervention "get better at regulating their emotions, they also start having friends, which in turn improves their emotion regulation in a positive cycle."

A key foundation of social competence is attachment, which focuses on the relationship between the child and the child's primary caregiver. We discuss attachment next.

DOI: 10.4324/9781003046455-2

Attachment: The Foundation of Emotional and Social Competence

What Is Attachment?

Attachment is a very special relationship. It begins in infancy and continues into adulthood. It influences all other relationships. Psychologists define it as a deep, enduring emotional bond between people. The person you are attached to is called an "attachment figure (AF)." This is a person you go to if you are upset. This person helps you feel safe and secure when they are around. Children live with an inherent tension between wanting to feel safe but wanting to explore and learn about their world. Attachment provides the solution to that tension. AFs are a "secure base" that makes children feel safe, so they can go exploring but are also people they can retreat to when they feel anxious, frightened, or hurt. Attachment is like a strong magnet that keeps children close to an adult who protects them.

Attachment is so important to children's well-being that government policies try to keep infants with their parents even when the parents are in drug rehab or incarcerated. These policies began after René Spitz compared infants in two different settings in 1952. One was a nursery for infants of mothers in jail. The infants had full access to their mothers in jail, and they developed normally. The second setting was a group home for infants whose mothers gave them up because they were too poor to feed them. These infants did nothing but lie in their cribs and rarely had any social interaction, but they were fed. Sadly, by the time these infants were a year old, they behaved bizarrely, such as silently huddling and rocking themselves, or screaming and crying if someone approached them. You can see René Spitz's films of these children on YouTube. These distressing videos helped convince people that infants should not be deprived of contact with an AF because attachment is a critical need in children. Attachment is important for children across all cultures. In fact, the early research on attachment occurred in many different countries from Scotland to Uganda.

Children attach to more than one person, but only a handful of people, usually parents and siblings and perhaps some other family members (e.g., grandparents, cousins, aunts, or uncles) or caregivers. These AFs form a hierarchy with one preferred person at the top. You can easily identify the primary AF – it is the person children go to first when upset, the one who most soothes them, and the one who causes the most upset when gone. Children may be comforted by other members of the hierarchy, but they prefer the primary AF. They may also prefer a different AF to play with. For example, mom might be the one they go to for comfort, but dad might be the one they go to for play.

Is Attachment Always Secure?

All typically developing children become attached, but their attachment can be *secure* or *insecure*. Psychologists can tell if a toddler is securely (vs. insecurely) attached by their behavior. This might surprise you, but it is not how loudly they cry or cling when the AF tries to leave. Instead, it is how they behave when their AF returns. *Securely* attached toddlers calm down immediately when the AF returns after being gone. They play contentedly when their AF is near and strongly show clear preference for the AF. In contrast, *insecurely* attached toddlers may either: (1) act like they do not notice that the AF returned after being gone or (2) cling to the AF but refuse to be comforted by the AF. Remember that not having a strong preference for an AF – going to anyone – is not typical and may signal an attachment problem. If you want to see how attachment works, ask a mother to go alone into a room in the house to quietly read a book. See how long before her young children move into the room. Securely attached children like to be near their AFs even while pursuing their own activities.

How Common Is Secure Attachment?

Roughly half of children (50–60%) are secure. These rates are generally similar across cultures, but may be higher in cultures (e.g., west African) where mothers and infants spend more time together. Whether a child is securely or insecurely attached tends to stay the same across childhood. However, a secure child can become insecure if there is a major life disruption such as divorce or increasing hours in childcare. It is possible, but less common, for an insecure child to become secure, for example, if family life stabilizes.

What Causes Secure Attachment?

Secure attachment is the result of the quality of interaction the AF has with a particular child. Across cultures, research has found that secure children have AFs who:

(a) cherish them and make sure the children (at any age) know that they are loved.
(b) are responsive to children's signals. If children cry, the AF comforts them. If they laugh, the AF smiles back. If they signal a need, the AF helps.
(c) are psychologically available. This does not mean that AFs are at children's beck-and-call all the time. If AFs are going about a task, such as making dinner, and the child wants to show them something, the AF quickly looks and admires, and then returns to making dinner. This kind of brief, but immediate, responsiveness teaches children that they can get the most important people in their world to respond to them and that they matter.

In contrast, insecure children have AFs who are insensitive and self-centered. They may behave like their children are a nuisance to them or deliberately try to irritate them. They may respond inconsistently (sometimes they respond, sometimes they don't) or only respond when their children's signals are extreme, like throwing a tantrum or getting kicked out of high school. Other AFs may be intrusive. This means they do things based on their own agenda, ignoring their children's agenda. For example, just when a child is absorbed in a toy, the AF says the child should try a different toy and exchanges it. This kind of behavior makes children feel helpless, unimportant, frustrated, and angry. Other AFs may be abusive, which makes their children feel frightened by the very people who should take care of them. This creates a terrible dilemma for children. Fortunately, there are interventions that can help parents learn to be more sensitive, which we will discuss in Chapter 11.

Children in low-income or historically marginalized families are more likely to be insecurely attached and have insensitive parents, perhaps due to family stress and risk factors linked to low income. However, secure attachment occurs despite risk factors when parents are sensitive. At the other extreme, high-income parents who are intrusive, or absent, may also have children with insecure attachment. For attachment, quality of parent–child interaction matters more than income or social status.

In addition to quality of parenting, attachment security is also affected by amount and quality of childcare. Children are less likely to be securely attached if they are in low-quality, unstable childcare and if they are in childcare for more than 10 hours per week. Childcare is stressful to children. Cortisol, a stress hormone, naturally peaks in the morning to wake you up and give you energy for the day, and then wanes in the evening to prepare you to sleep. However, children in childcare experience rising cortisol over the day instead of waning (Gunnar, 2021). Children who are in childcare at a young age may continue to have abnormal cortisol levels as adolescents, long after leaving childcare. Due to stress and feeling less secure, by age 3 children in childcare tend to have less self-control and more behavior problems, such as attention deficits, conflict, hyperactivity, aggression, and impulsivity. If parents limit children's amount of time in childcare and are especially sensitive, they can diminish but not eliminate the effects of childcare stress on their children. Some children with easy temperaments are less affected by childcare.

Siblings Are Attachment Figures

Most children (80% in the USA) have siblings. Other than attachment to parents or some other AF, children's first and deepest social relationships are with siblings. The sibling relationship is the longest of all relationships (it will outlast parent–child relationships). Siblings can be AFs who provide security to one another. However, siblings can have either close or conflicted relationships. Relationships begin when a new baby enters the home. How parents talk about the infant to older siblings influences the kind of relationship that develops. Some parents say "don't touch the baby, you might hurt him!" whereas others tell the older siblings "this is your baby" and teach them to read the signals of the infant, hold the infant safely, and empathize with the infant (e.g., "he's crying because he is lonely – can you talk to him?" or "look he's smiling at you – he loves you!"). Can you see how these two different approaches can result in positive or negative relationships over time? When parents teach siblings to serve and help each other, have fun together, build memories, and resolve conflict well, siblings are more likely to develop positive relationships.

The sibling relationship is rich soil for growing social skills and learning to regulate emotions. This is because sibling relationships tend to be the most conflicted of all relationships. This might surprise you, but sibling conflict, if it is not extreme, is *good for children*, because it provides opportunity to practice apologizing, forgiving, and moral reflection, as a training ground for moral character. Most sibling conflict is over possessions or space. *He took my toy! He ate my cookie!* Older siblings usually win such conflicts, but younger siblings may develop greater negotiation, compromise, and theory of mind skills (discussed below) that will serve them well in adulthood.

When parents need to intervene in order to help siblings use compromise successfully, it is important to use other-oriented induction (Chapter 4). This helps to train empathy in children and communicates that they are responsible for the way they treat others. Furthermore, sibling conflict is an opportunity to talk about emotions, which leads to greater emotional competence. For example, a parent might say "I know it makes you angry when he takes your stuff, but he is jealous because he wants to be able to do what you do. He looks up to you." This engenders empathy toward the sibling, better understanding of emotions (anger and jealousy), and ability to read others.

Why Does Attachment Matter?

Thousands of studies across many cultures have found that secure attachment is vitally important for at least three reasons.

1. Attachment is the foundation of emotional well-being, personality, and mental health. Secure children develop a happy, trusting core. Secure children also react more adaptively to stress. They are less likely to have ADHD symptoms, depression, anxiety, behavior disorders, and substance abuse. In contrast, insecure attachment mimics the symptoms of ADHD as it leads to anxiety, depression, and anger-based behavior problems.
2. Attachment is the foundation of social competence because it is where relationship skills are learned. Attachment influences how children get along in

the social world. Compared to insecure children, secure children have more harmonious friendships, more empathy, greater resistance to peer pressure, less aggression, and a stronger social support network. They have healthier marriages in adulthood.

3. Attachment is the foundation of self-esteem. Whether a child feels worthy of love, or not, comes from attachment relationships. Securely attached children learn that the *self* is valuable and worthy of love, and that *others* are trustworthy, responsive, and caring. In contrast, insecure children learn that they are not worthy of love and that others cannot be trusted to care for them consistently.

This is an amazing array of important outcomes! You can see why developing a secure attachment is one of the most important things a parent can do for a child. However, keep in mind that while secure attachment is an important asset, and insecure attachment is a risk factor, science is about probability, not certainty. Some insecure children will develop social competence. Let's discuss this next.

What Is Social Competence?

Social competence is defined as being effective in relationships and social situations. The official definition from the American Psychological Association (APA) is given in Box 2.1. More poetically, you can think of social competence as "moving *with* and moving *against* others." Psychologists call this prosocial and antisocial behavior. Socially competent children engage in prosocial behavior *with* others and refrain from antisocial behavior *against* others. Notice that these terms are about the *quality* of behavior, not *quantity* or how much you are social. That is, being prosocial does not mean being outgoing and being antisocial does not mean being shy. Jamal, in the opening vignette, is a quiet, shy boy who seldom volunteers answers in class, but pays attention and readily answers when his teacher calls on him. Jamal is prosocial toward his classmates and his teacher.

Box 2.1   Definition of Social Competence

The APA Dictionary of Psychology states that social competence is "effectiveness or skill in interpersonal relations and social situations, increasingly considered an important component of mental health. Social competence involves the ability to evaluate social situations and determine what is expected or required; to recognize the intentions of others; and to select social behaviors that are most appropriate for that given context. It is important to note, however, that what is required and appropriate for effective social functioning is likely to vary across settings."

Prosocial Behavior: What It Is and Why It Matters

Prosocial behavior *is any behavior intended to benefit others and promote harmonious relationships* – such as sharing, cooperating, helping, encouraging, complimenting, respecting, comforting, and defending others. It is *selfless* (compared to *selfish*) behavior. You can think of it as being "nice," but prosocial behavior goes beyond merely being nice because sometimes it requires assertion (e.g., standing up for someone else) or taking an unpopular, but moral, stance. Jamal, in the opening vignette, is a prosocial youth.

Prosocial behavior is an important asset for children because the more prosocial they are, the greater their own well-being and the greater the well-being of those around them, like peers, teachers, and family. Children who are prosocial tend to be happy, calm, and well-liked by others. Think about how good you feel when you've helped someone. Prosocial children also tend to earn higher grades and test scores at school because they take turns, listen, and stay on task (Bergin, 2018). Teachers enjoy teaching more when their students are kind and collaborative. Furthermore, prosocial children tend to be more resilient when faced with trauma or adversity. Prosocial behavior protects youth from delinquency, risky sexual behavior, substance use, depression, and emotional problems. When prosocial children enter adulthood, they are more likely to be successful in the workplace because they collaborate and show respect for others. Adults who work with children can help them become more prosocial. In later chapters we'll discuss how you can promote children's prosocial behavior.

Antisocial Behavior: What It Is and Why It Matters

The opposite of prosocial behavior, antisocial behavior, is moving *against* others. It is any behavior that harms others or disrupts the functioning of a social group – such as aggression, vandalism, delinquency, or hostile behavior. We'll focus on aggression here.

Aggression can be physical, verbal, or relational. Physical aggression is hitting, kicking, biting, and shoving. Verbal aggression is insulting, threatening, and name-calling. Social aggression is excluding others, spreading rumors, or damaging reputations (think "Mean Girls"). Both verbal and social aggression can occur online or in person. Children who use one type of aggression often use the other types as well. But this shifts with age, which we'll discuss below.

Aggression also varies by motive. *Instrumental aggression* is where one child harms another in order to get something they want, but not with the intent of hurting the other. For example, a 3-year-old may shove another child to get a ball, but not to deliberately hurt the other child. *Reactive aggression* is where a child counter-attacks someone who has attacked them; they are aggressive out

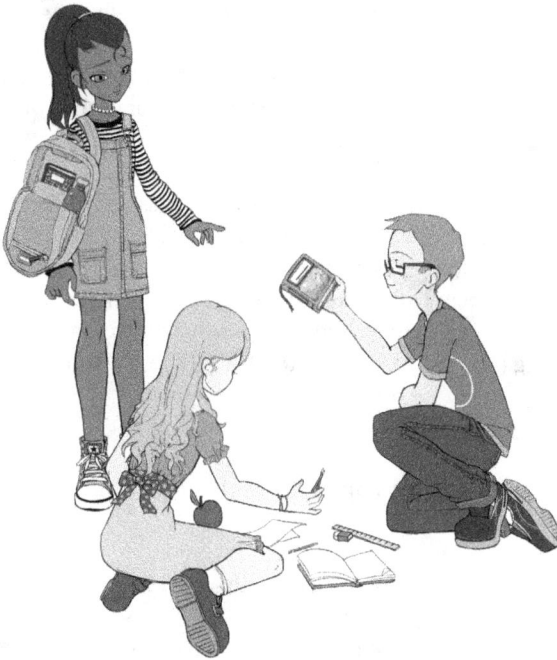

Figure 2.1 Prosocial behavior is valued across cultures as a core component of social competence.

of anger or frustration and may hit someone who hit them. *Bullying* is unprovoked, hostile aggression that is repeated toward someone with less power or status; the intent is to dominate, intimidate, humiliate, or harm the victim. The most common form of bullying is making fun of others or spreading rumors about them. Watch for examples of aggression you see in person or in the media and identify: (1) what the motive is and (2) whether it is physical, verbal, or relational aggression.

Most children are only occasionally aggressive, but about 5–15% are frequently aggressive. Being aggressive is a stable trait, meaning that young children who are more aggressive than their same-age peers are likely to stay that way into adulthood unless they receive intervention (e.g., Zych et al., 2020). Whether a child is more aggressive than others is *one of the most stable attributes* across ethnic/racial groups across countries. This is a problem because antisocial children tend to do more poorly in school from kindergarten through high school, although the effects are strongest in high school. They have attention problems, reading difficulties, lower Grade Point Averages (GPAs), and lower test scores. Antisocial children are also likely to be rejected by their peers, leading to either loneliness or becoming friends with other antisocial youth. Aggressive youth tend to become adults with substance use, poor jobs, periods of unemployment, marital conflict, divorce, and harsh parenting of their own children. They can get off this grim trajectory if they develop prosocial behavior, learn a valuable skill, and become part of a healthy social network.

Which children are most likely to be aggressive? Risk factors identified by research are listed in Box 2.2. Not everyone who has one of these risk factors will become aggressive, but the more risk factors someone has, the greater the likelihood. Furthermore, if someone has protective factors (e.g., religiosity, authoritative parents, secure attachment), they are less likely to become aggressive. Interventions for aggressive children typically involve training to improve quality of parenting (Van Goozen et al., 2022). You'll learn more about interventions in Chapters 8–11.

Box 2.2   Risk Factors for Aggression

1. Poor emotion regulation (easily angered).
2. Poor affective perspective-taking (see Chapter 1).
3. Insecure attachment.
4. Exposed to power assertive discipline from parents.
5. Low self-control.
6. Watch violent sexualized media.
7. Poor conflict resolution skills.
8. Long hours in childcare or self-care.
9. Parental divorce and/or conflict.

Shyness: What It Is and Why It Matters

Some children are outgoing and greet new people with enthusiasm. Others are shy, cautious, and hang back when meeting new people. This has nothing to do with whether they are prosocial or antisocial in their behavior. That is, a shy person may be very kind or mean. The same is true for a boisterous, outgoing person. Thus, both shy and outgoing children can be socially competent.

Shyness can be good, if it is not extreme. Shy, cautious behavior protects children from being aggressive or taking dangerous risks. Some children are "shy-sociable." This means they hang back from new people but are quite sociable with familiar people. Other children are "shy-non-sociable." This means they hang back even from familiar people. Being shy-sociable is not a problem because these children have friends. However, shy-non-sociable children are at risk for loneliness and rejection from peers. They may have high anxiety in typical social settings, like attending school.

How Does Social Competence Change with Age?

Just like emotional competence, your social competence should have improved dramatically since birth, becoming more sophisticated and complex. Babies are born with an innate tendency to be prosocial (see Chapter 3). It is so universal that at age 12 months, if a baby doesn't share with or try to help others, it is viewed as a sign of possible development problems. At the same time, toddlers can also be angry and throw tantrums, leading them to hit, bite, and kick others. This physical aggression tends to peak about age 2–3. Preschoolers are the most aggressive of any age, but their aggression is mostly intended to get something rather than harm others. For example, they may push someone off the slide so they can slide, not because they want to harm the other child. How to handle such aggression in toddlers is illustrated in Box 2.3.

Box 2.3 Toddler Case Study

Toddlers who do not have any words yet may bite another child to get what they want. This behavior is typical. However, once toddlers have words and can communicate effectively, they will decrease or stop biting others. Adults should respond differently depending on a toddlers' ability to talk. A biting toddler without words may be redirected to play with another toy. On the other hand, toddlers who bite in order to get a toy could be told that "We don't bite. It hurts others. Look, you made him cry. Can you bring him another toy to make him happy?" The way you address the situation should be different based on children's ability to use language, control their emotions, and understand others' feelings.

You may have noticed that shyness is common among preschoolers. They may hide behind their parent if a stranger tries to talk to them. By middle childhood, they become less shy. They also become less aggressive overall. But when they are aggressive, it is more likely to be verbal and social aggression rather than physical. By middle childhood, their prosocial skills have grown to the point that they may be asked to help tend younger siblings.

As children enter adolescence in middle school, there is a dip in prosocial behavior and a temporary rise in bullying. Adolescents tend to be less helpful or affectionate in the family. This will improve as they enter young adulthood. Prosocial behavior grows and antisocial behavior declines from adolescence into young adulthood. While a subset of adolescents may have a temporary surge in antisocial and delinquent behavior, most adolescents are not aggressive or delinquent.

Children's growing social competence is reflected in their play. Infants begin showing back-and-forth social play with adults, such as peek-a-boo, but the adult has to scaffold it. By age 2, toddlers play in "parallel" with other children. This means they play near each other with the same or similar toys, but without much interaction or sharing (Biddle et al., 2013). By age 4, children play make-believe games with rules and a common goal, such as playing "cooks" who serve food to others. In middle childhood through young adulthood, play gets more complex and may be competitive, such as organized sports or board games. We'll discuss the social milestones and skills associated with different ages in greater detail in Chapters 3–6.

In What Ways Do Individuals Differ in Social Competence?

While there are clear general age trends in the development of social competence, two children of the same age can differ in their level of social competence. One reason is that children vary in their emotional competence, which you learned about in Chapter 1. Three other reasons are: (1) their social cognition, (2) their self-control, and (3) their ability.

Social Cognition

"Cognition" refers to thinking. In every social situation, you are thinking about and interpreting your own and others' behavior. A theory called *Social Information Processing (SIP) Theory* (Dodge et al., 2022) suggests there are six steps in the way you think about social situations.

1. Perceiving social cues in other people's behavior ("My sister is scowling at me").
2. Giving meaning to the social cues ("She knows I took her cookie").
3. Getting specific about your goals in the situation ("I don't want to get in trouble").
4. Creating and visualizing responses ("I could smirk, but she'll tell Dad or I could apologize and maybe she won't tell Dad").
5. Choosing a response ("I'll apologize and say how hungry I was").
6. Enacting and evaluating the behavior ("I apologized and it worked; she didn't tell Dad").

Children differ in their SIP at an early age. Some have a hostile bias when reading others in Step 2. They may have a "chip on their shoulder," which means they expect others to be hostile. This tends to make them choose aggressive goals ("get her before she gets me"), so they are wary and aggressive towards others. On the other hand, you may know someone with "rose-colored glasses," which means they expect others to be prosocial, so they are polite and kind towards others. Can you see how your thoughts about others can influence social competence? Some interventions use SIP principles to help children become more socially competent by changing their anxious or aggressive thoughts (Santone et al., 2020). Interventions can happen along all six steps of SIP, sometimes addressing more than one step. For example, Step 1 is perceiving social cues in other people's behavior. One set of interventions teaches youth to think about several alternatives for other people's behavior. Let's say José bumps Tommy when walking to his seat. Tommy jumps to the conclusion that José wants to provoke him, but Tommy can be taught to consider alternative explanations like José did not see Tommy or José stumbled while walking. Which explanation is less likely to result in a fight?

The ability to understand your own mental states and the mental states of others is called "theory of mind." It refers to knowing that other people can have mental states – ideas, beliefs, intentions, and knowledge – that are different from your own, and being able to infer those mental states. Tommy needs to consider José's possible thoughts and whether they might not be hostile. You can think of it as the ability to read others' minds to some extent. For example, Reece hid in the closet to play with her mother's cell phone. Why did she hide? Because she could read her mother's mind well enough to know her mother did not want her to play with the phone.

Generally, children who have better people-reading skills are more prosocial and less antisocial. Children with skillful theory of mind skills in early childhood are later rated as more socially competent in middle childhood by their teachers (Devine et al., 2016; Weimer, 2020). However, it is possible for some children to use skillful theory of mind for antisocial reasons, such as using their skills to lie convincingly in order to get others in trouble.

Clearly, some children's social cognition is more accurate, whereas others' is more distorted. Where do these individual differences come from? They come from social experiences inside and outside the family. Children who are abused have a wariness toward others, being hypervigilant to any signals that they might be unsafe. Children who watch violent media tend to develop a "mean world" bias, expecting hostility from others. Children with insecure attachment to parents develop the belief that others are undependable or hostile. Children with depressed mothers tend to have difficulty reading others accurately and have lower social competence.

These individual differences among children can also come from biological abnormalities or learning differences (Campbell et al., 2015). For instance, the absence of certain genes on the 22nd chromosome is related to poor social cognition. This genetic condition may lead to: (1) difficulty reading others' emotions or their thoughts, (2) difficulty initiating social interaction, and (3) anxiety, ADHD, and autism spectrum disorder, which diminish social competence and disrupt relationships.

Self-Control

Children of the same age can also differ in their level of social competence due to differences in self-control. Self-control is the ability to inhibit impulses and regulate your thoughts, behaviors, and emotions. It helps you stay focused on a task despite distractions, obey rules, be patient, and pay attention. It helps you inhibit impulses in the moment in order to attain bigger goals. Resisting something right now in order to get something in the long-run is called "delay of gratification." For example, you might resist playing a videogame right now in order to study so that you can become a more competent professional. Self-control is related to emotion regulation, which is control of your emotions. Self-control is called for many times each day, for adults as well as young children.

Whether a child is high or low in self-control for their age tends to be quite stable across childhood. This means that a 4-year-old with good self-control (for a preschooler) is likely to become a 20-year-old with good self-control (for a young adult). These differences have important consequences. Children with good self-control for their age tend to have higher grades and test scores in school and finish more years of college education. They are less likely to use alcohol and other drugs. They also are more prosocial and less aggressive. They are more cooperative with others and liked better by teachers and classmates.

Why do some children have better self-control for their age? One reason is they have better *executive function,* which is a brain-based process that allows us to shift our focus of attention and inhibit behavior (Devine et al., 2016). It is what allows you to keep a long-term goal in mind while you process what is happening in the moment. It is also what allows you to plan, focus, and flexibly shift from thinking about one thing to another. It is the foundation of theory of mind.

Self-control aspects of executive function are built through experience. You can build self-control over time by practicing it. However, keep in mind that if you overly stress self-control, it can fail from fatigue. Self-control is like a muscle – you can only exert so much self-control before it fails just like you can only lift so much weight before your muscles give way. That is why you need to occasionally take a break from a task that demands your self-control.

Two social experiences that build self-control are: (1) religiosity and (2) parenting. Children tend to have more self-control if they are active in religion (perhaps because most religions emphasize self-mastery). Children also tend to have more self-control if they have secure attachment to parents who monitor them, restrict media use, are warm but demanding, and use respectful discipline, which you'll learn more about in Chapter 4.

Ability

Children's abilities and disabilities – such as intelligence, learning disabilities, neuro-diversity, or congenital disorders – influence their development of social competence (Corbett et al., 2016). Children with disabilities may be given interventions such as academic support, an alternative educational environment, therapy, medicine, or adaptive technology in order to support their social competence. Interview Box 2.4 shows how a former middle school teacher helped students with different abilities develop social competence.

Box 2.4   Interview with an Educator

Lucy is now a college professor, but used to be a middle school teacher.

How is social competence related to learning differences?

Thought processes play a crucial role in the development and enactment of social competence. Context and culture influence our thought processes. Hence, context and culture influence the way we enact social competence. A standard of behavior from one context is different in another context. When children interact with adults, they have to be mindful about the norms and ways of behaving. This is different when they interact with peers.

How have you promoted the social competence of children with learning differences?

When I taught middle school, I focused on language and literacy as tools for students to use when enacting social competence. This relates to my comment about thought processes. When students learn ways of thinking about other people through stories and narratives, this enriches their knowledge of behavior, which can then affect their social competence. For instance, I used books as a springboard to deal with bullying or empathy. Specific strategies include:

1. Use literature to understand people's ways of behaving.
2. Model social competence.
3. Reflect on one's behavior.
4. Share stories that demonstrate social competence.
5. Reinforce gradual approximation of behavior. That is, shape children's behavior through small steps.

Peers helped in two ways. First, I explicitly pointed out in peers the specific behavior to emulate. Second, the students with learning differences
could practice the behavior with peers.

In What Ways Do Groups Differ in Social Competence?

The specific behaviors that might be considered socially competent differ
depending on gender, culture, and ethnicity/race (Collie, 2020).

Gender

Aggression is one of the most robust gender differences. Research consistently finds that boys are more aggressive than girls, on average, across cultures
(Tremblay et al., 2018). There is a "mean girls" myth that girls are more socially
aggressive than boys. This is not true; boys are more aggressive in all ways,
including social. However, when girls are aggressive, it is more often social
aggression, rather than physical.

You might assume that girls are more prosocial than boys on average, but
this is not clear. Some studies find that girls are more prosocial and some find
boys and girls are similarly prosocial. Usually when studies find girls are more
prosocial, the research uses self- or teacher-report rather than observation. So, it
may be a bias in reporting; that is, people think girls are more prosocial, so they
report them as more prosocial.

Research on whether boys or girls are more shy is mixed. During the preschool
years, girls may be a little more socially anxious and withdrawn than boys. But
there is little evidence of gender differences at later ages. Unfortunately, when
boys are shy, they are more likely to be rejected by peers than are girls.

Culture and Ethnicity

In Chapter 1, you learned that different cultures have rules about what emotions can be expressed when and to whom. Cultures also have different expectations, rules, values, and norms for children's social behavior. Some cultures
view boisterous children as behavior problems and shy children as especially
mature, but other cultures may have the opposite view. Some cultures view pursuing individual well-being as more important than collective well-being, but
other cultures have the opposite view. Such variations in culture lead to different
expectations of what social competence looks like (Weimer, 2020).

Within a country, there can be many different subcultures. It is important to
remember as you work with children that they may share some aspects of your

culture, but may also have different expectations, beliefs, and social behaviors from yours. For example, a teacher thought a girl in her class was not very bright because she did not raise her hand or call out answers in class. The girl, Garuka, was an immigrant from an African culture that viewed such behavior as rude and arrogant. In fact, Garuka was very bright; she spoke multiple languages and was a mathematics whiz. Misinterpretation of the social behavior of children who have cultural differences from teachers may partly explain why more males are in Special Education and more African Americans are in alternative schools (Perzigian, 2018). Their culture may be different from teachers who tend to be female, middle class, and European American. It is important to avoid false assumptions that could lead to undermining children's well-being.

On the other hand, there are many similarities across cultures. For example, prosocial behavior is highly valued across cultures (see Figure 2.1). Yet, prosocial behavior may be expressed in different ways across cultures (Biddle et al., 2013). In Garuka's culture, socially competent parents quietly wait at the classroom door until the teacher invites them to step into the room. In another student's culture, the parents may walk right in and shake the teacher's hand. Both have prosocial intentions to honor the teacher by doing what is "polite" in their culture.

Contexts

Which behaviors are considered socially competent can vary by the context (see Box 2.5). You probably behave differently when talking with your boss than when talking with your friend because the "social rules" of the context are different. Children have to learn what behavior is acceptable in different contexts. For example, yelling to a teammate may be socially acceptable on a soccer field but not in a classroom. Scoffing at a friend's comment may be socially acceptable but not scoffing at a principal who is reprimanding you (Biddle et al., 2013; Collie, 2020). Children are expected to act differently if they are with a psychologist (sit and talk about feelings), versus with a nurse (lay still and allow them to examine you), versus with their peers at a park (run and shout).

Box 2.5 Context Case Study

Socially competent youth behave in ways that fit social expectations for the context. For example, in a school context, socially competent youth behave in ways that fit school expectations. This might mean that they use formal English, participate in groups activities, talk about school events like sports competitions, adhere to clothing expectations, and follow classroom rules. In contrast, in social contexts with friends outside of school, socially competent youth may be more boisterous, use slang, dress casually, share hobbies, and show their personalities with less constraint. In both settings, youth manage how they appear to peers and adults.

Children's behavior is more accepted when it matches what is "normal" in a context. Children who behave aggressively in a highly aggressive classroom are more likely to be accepted by peers in that class. In contrast, children who behave aggressively in a classroom with little aggression may be rejected by peers in that class.

Chapter Summary

Social competence is separate from emotional competence, yet they are tightly related. Social competence grows in complexity with age. However, two children of the same age can have different levels of social competence. Socially competent children are high in prosocial behavior and low in antisocial behavior. Children's level of aggression tends to be quite stable across childhood. Shyness does not affect whether a child is socially competent unless it is extreme even with familiar others. Individual differences in social competence have important consequences for children's long-term well-being. Those differences are partly driven by children's social cognition as outlined by the SIP model, including theory of mind, and their self-control. They may also be driven by biologically based disabilities.

There are some differences in social behaviors between boys and girls, with aggression being the most pronounced – on average, boys are more aggressive than girls. The behaviors that are considered socially competent may vary across cultures and contexts, such as school, home, community, or peer group. Adults from a dominant culture who interact with children from a marginalized culture must take this into account when evaluating social competence. Parents, teachers, librarians, school administrators, psychologists, therapists, behavioral technicians, social workers, and child life specialists can increase a child's social competence. We'll discuss how in Chapters 3–11. The SIP model is helpful as an intervention tool to help children with social competence.

Suggestions for Further Rereading

Fiske, S., &Taylor, S. E. (2021). *Social cognition: From brains to culture*. Sage.

Del Prette, Z., & Del Prette, A (2021). *Social competence and social skills: A theoretical and practical guide*. Springer.

Tierney, J., Green, E., Dowd, T, & McGrady, K. (2022). *Teaching social skills to youth: An easy-to-follow guide to teaching 196 basic to complex life skills*. 4th ed. Boys Town Press.

References

Bergin, C. (2018). *Designing a prosocial classroom: Fostering collaboration in students from pre-K-12 with the curriculum you already use.* Norton.

Biddle, K. A., García-Nevarez, A., Henderson, W., Valero-Kerrick, A. (2013). *Early childhood education: Becoming a professional.* Sage.

Campbell, L., McCabe, L., Melville, J., Strutt, P., & Schall, U. (2015). Social cognition dysfunction in adolescents with 22q11.2 deletion syndrome (velo-cardio-facial syndrome): Relationship with executive functioning and social competence/functioning. *Journal of Intellectual Disability Research, 59*(9), 845–859.

Collie, R. (2020). The development of social and emotional competence at school: An integrated model. *International Journal of Behavioral Development, 44*(1), 76–87.

Corbett, B.A., Key, A., Qualls, L., Fecteau, S., Newsom, C., Coke, C., & Yoder, P. (2016). Improvement in social competence using a randomized trial of a theatre intervention for children with autism spectrum disorder. *Journal of Autism and Developmental Disorders, 46*(2), 658–672.

Devine, R.T., White, N., Ensor, R., & Hughes, C. (2016). Theory of mind in middle childhood: Longitudinal associations with executive function and social competence. *Developmental Psychology, 52*(5) 758–771.

Dodge, K. A., Bai, Y., Godwin, J., Lansford, J. E., Bates, J. E., Pettit, G. S., & Jones, D. (2022). A defensive mindset: A pattern of social information processing that develops early and predicts life course outcomes. *Child Development, 93*(4), e357–e378. https://doi.org/https://doi.org/10.1111/cdev.13751

Gunnar, M. R. (2021). Forty years of research on stress and development: What have we learned and future directions. *American Psychologist, 76*(9), 1372–1384.

Perzigian, A. (2018). Social competence in urban alternative schools. *Pennsylvania GSE Perspectives on Urban Education, 15*(1), 1–13.

Santone, E., Crothers, L.M., Kolbert, J.B., & Miravalle, J. (2020). Using social information processing theory to counsel aggressive youth. *Journal of School Counseling. 18*(18), 1–34.

Tremblay, R. E., Vitaro, F., & Côté, S. M. (2018). Developmental origins of chronic physical aggression: A bio-psycho-social model for the next generation of preventive interventions. *Annual Review of Psychology, 69*, 383–407.

van Goozen, S., Langley, K., & Hobson, C. W. (2022). Childhood antisocial behavior: A neurodevelopmental problem. *Annual Review of Psychology, 73*, 353–377.

Weimer, A. A. (2020). Theory of mind and social competence among school-age Latino children. *Early Child Development and Care. 190*(6), 902–910.

Zych, I., Ttofi, M. M., Llorent, V. J., Farrington, D. P., Ribeaud, D., & Eisner, M. P. (2020). A longitudinal study on stability and transitions among bullying roles. *Child Development, 91*(2), 527–545.

Chapter 3

Social and Emotional Competence in Early Childhood (Birth to Age 5)

Issac, a 2-year-old, and his father are at the grocery store. After bagging their groceries, Dad says "Let's go." But Issac says "No!" (his favorite word) and tries to reach candy from a display case. Dad says "No candy right now. Its time to go." Issac crumples to the floor, sobbing. When Dad tries to pick him up and comfort him, Issac arches his back, kicks, and sobs even louder. Dad looks appalled. He is embarrassed and feels helpless, but also feels compassion for his distraught son. Nothing Dad does seems to help.

Is this normal behavior for toddlers, or does Issac lack emotion regulation skills? What should his father do? In this chapter, you will learn the answer to these questions as we discuss development of social–emotional competence during early childhood.

Early childhood refers to the period from birth to about age 5. In this book, we will use the common terms "infant" for children who are 0–12 months old, "toddler" for 1- to 2-year-olds, and "preschooler" for 3- to 5-year-olds. Remarkable changes occur in children during this 5-year span. They transform from completely immobile infants to crawling, then toddling, then running on their own two feet. They also transform from communicating only through emotions and gestures (e.g., cries, smiles), to cooing and babbling, to one-word statements, to full conversations! The progress is amazing.

Development of Emotional Competence in Early Childhood

As soon as they are born, infants communicate through emotions to adults who take care of them. They might cry to say very different things like "Feed me," "I'm tired," and "I don't like my bath." They might laugh or smile to say "I like it when Daddy smiles at me" or "I like this food." Within a few years, infants will use language to communicate the same messages.

DOI: 10.4324/9781003046455-3

Table 3.1 Basic and Social Emotions

Early basic emotions	Later complex social emotions
Interest	Envy
Happiness	Embarrassment
Sadness	Shame
Anger	Guilt
Disgust	Pride
Fear	

Basic and Social Emotions

Infants express a few *basic emotions* at birth. Walk into a hospital newborn nursery, and you will see infants clearly express anger as the nurse weighs them or gives them a bath. You will also see them looking about with wide-eyed interest. The basic emotions that newborns express include interest, happiness, sadness, anger, disgust, and fear (see Table 3.1). At 4–6 weeks of age, infants typically give their first social smile, expressing happiness at seeing a friendly face looming over them. Around 4 months of age, they begin to laugh in response to tickling or peek-a-boo games.

Between 1 and 3 years, toddlers will begin to express "social" emotions like envy, embarrassment, shame, guilt, and pride. These emotions come a little later than basic emotions because they develop as toddlers come to understand their relationships with others. For example, if you catch toddlers sneaking a treat they are not supposed to have, they may quickly hide it and show guilt (e.g., lowered eyes with averted gaze, collapsed body posture). Social emotions are important for helping children learn to follow the norms of their family. For example, guilt motivates children to mend harm they have done. Pride motivates them to achieve things that their family values. Shame motivates them to abide by family expectations. These emotions continue to be important throughout life. For example, embarrassment makes you hurry so you do not walk into class late.

Emotion Regulation

Infants are born with a few tools to control their emotions. For example, when infants feel over-stimulated, they will suck the inside of their cheeks or shut their eyes. (Many adults mistakenly think they are asleep, but their furrowed brows may indicate they are not asleep.) Toddlers have techniques like sucking a thumb or cuddling with a blanket or stuffed animal. However, young children often need the help of adults to regulate their emotions. For example, an adult may cuddle, rock, or "shush" the child. This is called *co-regulation* because the adult and child together are regulating the child's emotions.

Young children gradually learn to regulate their emotions on their own by growing up inside a circle of caring adults who co-regulate with them. By the time they are preschoolers, they can use some coping strategies on their own (see Box 1.1). For example, they may distract themselves when they feel sad. However, preschoolers tend to engage in less constructive strategies (e.g., crying or kicking) more often than older children. Preschoolers also become more capable of faking their emotions, but their skill is not as good as it will be when they are older. For example, they are better at exaggerating rather than stifling an emotion, such as loudly wailing when they do not get a candy they want. They may even wait to wail until a parent is watching. That's pretty good emotion regulation!

Emotion Regulation and Attachment

Starting in infancy, children learn emotion regulation from their attachment figures (AFs) during routine activities such as feeding, bathing, and playing. Imagine that a toddler is sitting in a chair with his father. The father tickles him. The toddler laughs so hard he can barely catch his breath. The father backs off to let him calm down. Then the father swoops in and tickles him again. The toddler again laughs so hard he is gasping for breath. Again, this sensitive father backs off and waits until the toddler has calmed down. Thousands of repeated experiences like this will alter the toddler's networks in his brain, resulting in a brain that can control intense emotions. Now imagine a different father. This second father does not back off to let his toddler calm down, but instead overstimulates him so much that the toddler shifts from laughing intensely to crying. This second toddler may develop an angry emotional core and poor regulation if his father continues to be intrusive and insensitive to his child's emotions.

Insecure children have a history of parents who are inconsistent, insensitive, or hostile toward them. For example, parents may ignore subtle signs of distress until the child has a full-blown tantrum. Then, they finally notice their child's distress and, too late, attempt to soothe the child, or they harshly punish the child for being distressed (which only makes the child more distressed). Across thousands of emotional events over several years, these insecure children learn to have a rapid rise of intense emotions in order to attract their parents' inconsistent help, or they learn to squelch emotions to escape their parents' hostility. Neither pattern leads to constructive coping. Over time, such children increasingly come to feel anxious, angry, or depressed. They may become either emotionally needy and clingy toward others or detached and unfeeling in order to avoid emotional closeness.

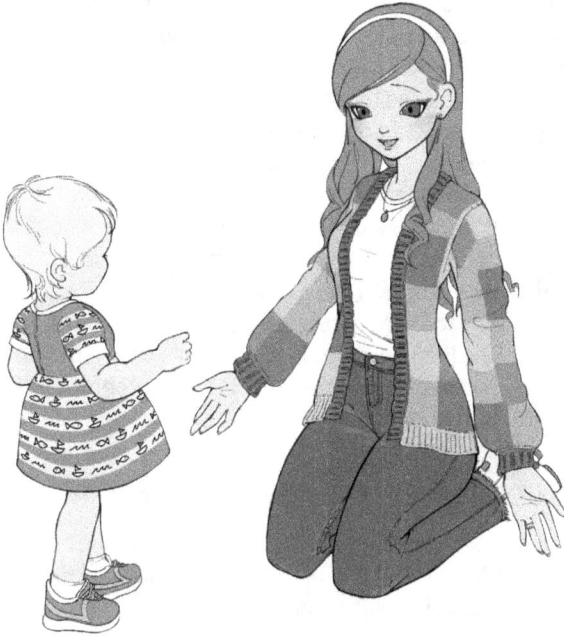

Figure 3.1 Secure attachment is foundational to both social and emotional competence.

In contrast, securely attached children are more likely to have good emotion regulation. Because their parents are sensitive, the children learn that others will help them cope with their emotions, and in the process they learn constructive coping strategies (see Figure 3.1).

Tantrums

Have you heard the term "terrible twos"? Anger is apparent in infants as young as 4 months. (You will see this if you try holding their arms down while they are in a high chair or stop them in the middle of play so you can change a diaper.) From 4 months to 2 years of age, anger, fussiness, and irritability steadily increase. Anger may increase because adults increasingly say "no!" to toddlers who innocently play in dangerous or destructive ways, such as pulling the tail of a dog. As a result, tantrums are common in toddlers. Fortunately, negativity decreases from age 2 to age 5 as toddlers learn to control their emotions.

Merely being angry or crying loudly over being hurt is not the same thing as a tantrum. Tantrums are defined as big emotions that are out of proportion for the situation and involve unreasonable behavior, like throwing yourself on the ground and kicking. A child who howls because she tripped on the sidewalk and skinned her knee is not having a tantrum; that is a reasonable response. However, a child who howls and throws himself on the floor at the grocery store because his father said he could not have candy could be having a tantrum; that is an unreasonable response.

Tantrums emerge around age 16 months and peak around 18–21 months. It is not unusual for toddlers to have a tantrum once a day, but by age 2, they should become less frequent. The worst is typically over by age 2, so it would be more accurate to say "the terrible ones" rather than "the terrible twos." Keep in mind that even older preschoolers may occasionally have a tantrum if they are tired, stressed, or hungry. Preschoolers might have tantrums once a month rather than daily. Issac is likely to soon outgrow tantrums in the grocery store if his parents are sensitive and responsive to him.

Reading Others' Emotions (Affective Perspective-Taking)

In Chapter 1, you learned about "affective perspective-taking" or the ability to read others' emotions. Young children have two tools that help them read others' emotions: emotional contagion and social referencing.

Emotional Contagion

In Chapter 1, you learned that emotional contagion occurs when the emotions of one person trigger similar emotions in another. This begins in infancy and continues across the life span. It may surprise you, but in the first hours of life newborns can mimic others' facial expressions and can tell one emotion from another (such as anger from surprise). They tend to pay particular attention to the eye region. Try it out! If you are face-to-face with a calm, alert, full-term newborn, stick out your tongue, or look very surprised. Within a few moments, the infant will likely imitate you. (Their response will be a little inconsistent and muted because they do not yet have full neurological control over facial muscles.)

Infants may "catch" our emotions, but do they really understand what they mean? Their reactions suggest that they do. For example, if an infant sees you looking sad, the infant may look away or suck their cheek, which are forms of self-soothing for negative emotions. On the other hand, if you look very happy, they may open their eyes wide and kick excitedly. In addition, social referencing suggests that they know what emotions mean.

Social Referencing

Social referencing refers to children reading others' emotional expressions as a guide for how they should respond to a situation they do not fully understand.

You will notice social referencing emerging between 6 and 10 months of age. It increases in importance over the next year so that toddlers will not approach something unknown and potentially scary (e.g., a stranger or a vacuum cleaner) until the parents' emotions signal that it is safe to approach. You can see how this skill is useful for young children's survival. For example, when a parent takes a toddler to the doctor's office, the toddler will intensely watch the parents' face for information about whether this is a safe or a scary place. If the parent smiles at the doctor, the toddler is more likely to interact in a friendly way with the doctor. In contrast, if the parent looks worried, the toddler is more likely to back away and resist the doctor. Thus, if you work with young children, it is helpful to recruit the parent to convey to their child that you are a safe person to approach.

Talk About Emotions

As they learn to talk, most young children label basic emotions as follows:

- About age 2: Use the emotion labels *happy* and *sad.*
- About age 3: Use more common emotion labels like *angry, scared,* and *surprised.*
- About age 5: Use as many common emotion labels as adults use, but continue to learn labels for less-common emotions into adulthood (Woodard et al., 2022).

Being able to label emotions helps young children understand causes and consequences of emotions. They begin talking about causes around age 3. For example, a 3-year-old boy told his mother, "Alan happy! I bring puppy" after giving his baby brother his favorite toy dog. By age 4, children know what emotions are typical of common situations (e.g., being angry if someone takes your toy). They also know that people may have different emotions about the same experience (e.g., some children are happy to jump in a puddle, but others are disgusted). By age 5, but seldom younger, children understand that you are more likely to forgive them if they express guilt, indicating they understand the social purpose of guilt (Tan et al., 2022).

Development of Social Competence in Early Childhood

In Chapter 2, you learned about attachment and that socially competent children engage in more prosocial, and less antisocial, behavior. Let's see how these develop in early childhood.

Attachment

Attachment can be secure or insecure. You can tell if a young child is secure by whether they are readily calmed by their AF when they are distressed and whether they show a clear preference for the AF. Box 3.1 illustrates what that may look like for two infants. Infants come pre-programmed to seek attachment relationships. While younger infants do not seem to mind being handed from person to person, starting around 9 months, infants will cry when an AF leaves them. This is called "separation distress." They also begin to be wary of strangers; this wariness peaks at about 12–24 months. Thus, it is *healthy and normal* for toddlers to cry when an AF leaves them with a babysitter. Separation distress then wanes, so that 3-year-olds may be alright with some separation, especially if their secondary AFs are around. For example, Dad may be able to leave a preschooler at home (a familiar setting) with an older sibling (a secondary AF) without the preschooler protesting. Around 4 years of age, many children are ready to go to preschool without a parent. In most countries with formal schooling, children begin to attend school away from their AF around ages 4–6.

Box 3.1   Attachment Case Study

Bruno (age 2 months) and Robbie (age 20 months) are cousins. Toddler Robbie often falls and starts crying. If a stranger picks him up, he will not calm down. But if his mother picks him up, he will calm right down as though he feels "I'm safe now. The person I trust to take care of me is here." If Robbie's grandmother picks him up, he will calm down. But if Mom is also in the room, he'll cry even louder until Grandmother hands him over to Mom. He clearly prefers Mom over Grandmother.

Robbie also toddles more excitedly toward his dad than to anyone else. Dad scoops him up, throws him in the air, tickles his tummy, turns him upside down, and then hugs him. If Robbie gets an "owie" during such rough-and-tumble play, he leaves Dad to get comfort from Mom. If Mom is not in the room, Robbie is readily comforted by Dad.

Dad and Grandmother are both high in Robbie's attachment hierarchy, but Mom is at the top. Mom feels a little jealous that Robbie enjoys playing with Dad more; Dad and Grandmother feel a little jealous that Robbie calms down better for Mom. But they are all glad that Robbie feels security from them, and that he is developing a healthy social and emotional core.

In contrast, the 2-month-old Bruno does not seem to care who holds him – doting cousins, aunts, uncles, parents, and neighbors. However,

---

they have noticed that Bruno has begun to turn his head toward his mothers' voice, to calm more readily with her, and to smile a little more for her. She loves it! Both Robbie's and Bruno's parents are falling more deeply in love with their child (parents get attached too)!

Prosocial Behavior

Infants come into the world prepared to be kind, empathic, and help others. How do we know this, given that infants can't talk or move? Scientists study infants' pupil dilation. Infants' pupils dilate, indicating anxious distress, when they see someone in need of help but then relax when help is given to the needy other. As soon as they become mobile, toddlers will actively try to help others. For example, if you drop something, they will pick it up for you even if they have to climb over an obstacle to do so. If they see someone cry, they will try to comfort them – perhaps bringing their own blankie or comfort toy to the crying person. There are lovely videos on YouTube of toddlers being prosocial (search for "Warneken, toddlers, prosocial").

Interestingly, the nearly universal impulse to be prosocial among infants begins to be less universal around age 2–3 (Martin & Olson, 2015). Toddlers begin to be more self-interested. They are more likely to help others who have helped them, or to share something they do not like as much, or to use sharing as a tool to get something they want. Although they become more selective, when they are helpful they are more effective. For example, a 4-year-old can effectively soothe a crying baby, whereas a 2-year-old might just pile toys on top of the baby.

The nearly universal impulse to be prosocial also transforms into individual differences in early childhood. That is, some children become more prosocial than others. These individual differences tend to persist across childhood, meaning that by ages 2–3, children who are more prosocial than others tend to stay that way (Romano et al., 2010). One study even found that preschoolers who shared more than others were also more generous in their 30s (Eisenberg et al., 2014). That's a remarkable span of time!

These individual differences in prosocial behavior have important consequences. In Chapter 2, you learned that children who are more prosocial are happier and liked better by others. This starts early; by 3 months of age, infants prefer prosocial others. When preschoolers are asked who they "like a lot" or most want to play with, the primary attribute of well-liked playmates is being prosocial. Prosocial preschoolers also tend to develop better early reading and math skills, perhaps because they are pleasant to interact with at home or in preschool classrooms.

What leads to some children becoming more prosocial than other children? There are at least four factors identified by research:

1. Secure attachment. Sensitive and responsive parents model kindness and meet their children's emotional needs, which frees their children to meet others' needs.
2. Emotional competence. Children who read other's emotions well and who can regulate their own emotions have more empathy.
3. Praise. Children who are praised for prosocial behavior tend to behave more prosocially, particularly if the praise comes from an adult with whom they have a warm relationship.
4. Practice. Children need opportunities to practice being prosocial toward others. This can include tasks in the family or preschool. Ideally, prosocial behavior becomes a well-worn habit.

Implications of this research are that if you work with young children, resist responding so quickly to a need that the children do not get a chance to respond. Accept their offers of help, even if inconvenient. For example, if someone drops an object, allow children to pick it up, and praise them for being good helpers, rather than stepping in to pick it up yourself.

Antisocial Behavior

Toddlers show aggression as soon as they are mobile; they will snatch, bite, and hit. There is a steady increase in aggression from age 1 to 3. *Three-year-olds are the most aggressive of any age group.* However, recall from Chapter 2 that there are different types and motives for antisocial behavior. Aggression in young children is *physical, instrumental* and short-lived. In fact, you may see toddlers in an angry fight over a toy who sit and play with each other a few minutes later, or the aggressor may even comfort the victim (Hay et al., 2011). *Instrumental aggression at this age is normal*; it does not foretell later problems.

Toddlers' aggression decreases once they develop good verbal skills, emotion regulation, and better theory of mind (or mind-reading) skills. Thus, by kindergarten, children are less aggressive than preschoolers (Vlachou et al., 2011). However, children's growing verbal ability also allows them to begin to replace physical with verbal aggression.

These are typical age trends, but individual children can differ in aggression. Preschoolers who are highly social tend to be *both* more prosocial and more antisocial. This is because they have more social interactions with other children and because they do not yet have strong social skills some interactions will be positive and some negative. As they grow in middle childhood, these highly social children will tend to specialize as predominantly prosocial or antisocial depending on their experiences. For this reason, you will want to redirect and instruct young children when they are aggressive. Interview Box 3.2 discusses how a coach works with children and their parents to find ways to build social skills.

In Chapter 1, you learned that children who have severe and chronic anti-social behavior for their age have "externalizing disorders." This is to distinguish antisocial behavior from anxiety and depression, which are "internalizing disorders." Young children with serious externalizing disorders may be diagnosed with *oppositional defiant disorder* (ODD), which is often a precursor to a diagnosis of *CD* as they get older. In Table 1.1, you may have noticed that part of externalizing disorders is impulsivity and hyperactivity. Aggression is commonly "comorbid" (meaning it goes together) with ADHD; about half of children with ADHD are also aggressive (Saylor & Amann, 2016). The most powerful risk factors for developing ODD are family dysfunction (see Chapter 1).

Theory of Mind

One of the most remarkable developments from age 3 to 5 is emergence of theory of mind, which was described in Chapter 2. The seed of the ability to read others' minds appears in infants. As young as 4 months, they will follow your gaze to see what you are interested in (Heyes, 2016). They will wait to reach for something out of reach until you are looking at them, so that you will know they want it. This indicates that they expect you to read their intent. If they see you look at an object with interest, but then pick up a different object, they will show surprise. One fun way scientists assess toddlers' ability to infer what you want is by having a bowl full of toy frogs and ducks. The scientist pulls only toy frogs from the bowl. Then, the bowl is removed and two bowls – one of only frogs and one of only ducks – is put in its place. The scientist then extends her hand between the two bowls. Toddlers with theory of mind will hand the scientist a frog! By age 3, children's theory of mind skills allow them to tease others. For example, Henry may pick up his brother's ball, look him in the eye, and then run away. When his brother chases him to get it back, Henry laughs with joy because he got just the reaction he wanted.

Box 3.2   Interview with a Parent Coach

Linda is a development specialist and parent coach.

How did you learn about social–emotional competence in children?

I learned in college in my BA and MA programs. I also did research on how to support a child's social–emotional competence. All professionals who work with children should understand these competencies. Children need them to develop in settings without adults. A child who lacks these skills will find it harder to reach other developmental milestones. Some children will need explicit teaching in social settings. However, many parents do not know they need to model and teach it. Some parents do not have these skills themselves. Part of my job is to help children learn social–emotional skills. I also teach parents how to teach their children these skills.

How do you help children and parents?

I work with children who lack these skills. I help them or teach their parents to help them socialize in various settings through play and interactions with peers and caregivers. I help them have positive interactions with toy exchanges, gaining joint attention, communicating wants and needs verbally and non-verbally. Culture should always be considered when measuring social competencies. However, it isn't always considered. Diagnosing children for disorders such as oppositional defiance, autism, or anxiety should always include a cultural component.

Development of the Self in Early Childhood

In Chapter 2, you learned that attachment influences social and emotional development. It also influences self-control and personality.

Self-Control

Young children are not yet skilled in self-control, but they make a lot of progress in the first 5 years of life. Self-control appears by the end of the first year. In the second year, children have the ability to obey caregivers and follow rules without a parent controlling them, such as "don't pull the dog's tail." One way that self-control is measured in young children is with the "marshmallow" task. Children are brought into a room and offered a marshmallow, but with a choice: They can eat one marshmallow right now, or if they wait a few minutes, they can have two. (You can watch a variety of these experiments on YouTube; search *Stanford Marshmallow Experiment*). By age 3, preschoolers can wait longer than toddlers. Similarly, when asked not to touch a tempting toy, 90% of toddlers cannot resist for more than 30 seconds, but 65% of 3-year-olds can (Friedman et al., 2011).

Children of the same age differ in self-control. One preschooler might wait several minutes, whereas another might wait less than a minute for a marshmallow. These individual differences in self-control are surprisingly stable. This means that a 3-year-old who can wait several minutes is likely to become an adult who has good self-control. These individual differences in preschool predict many important outcomes, such as later school success and health, including obesity (Schlam et al., 2013).

Personality and Identity

Next, we'll discuss temperament, which appears early in life and, with attachment, forms the basis of later personality.

Temperament

Temperament refers to the intensity and pattern of our reactions to the world around us. Psychologists do not fully agree on what traits are part of temperament, but most definitions include four components.

1. Activity (how much you move).
2. Negative emotionality (how easily you become irritated, disgusted, angry, or scared and how intense your emotions are).
3. Behavioral inhibition (how cautious and wary you are of novel things). In the social realm, this is called shyness.
4. Effortful control (how well you control your attention and impulses and resist distractions).

Temperament is identifiable by 4 months of age, but this does not mean it is necessarily inborn or genetically based. Attachment effects have already set in by then. By infancy, biology (e.g., pattern of brain response) is shaped by social experience like attachment. The godmother of attachment research, Mary Ainsworth, found that secure attachment is primarily driven by parent behavior and that a child's temperament makes only a small or no contribution. There may be some components of temperament that are heritable, but even those are influenced by children's social experiences. For example, many shy, inhibited children will outgrow it, but others will become *more* inhibited if they have parents who anxiously hover over them or are excessively critical. The personality traits you develop depend on the environment you are raised in. This is why temperament may not be stable for individual children. The first two components – activity and negativity – are more stable across childhood than behavioral inhibition and effortful control.

Some temperament traits are assets and some are risk factors. Negative emotionality and low effortful control are risk factors for later drug use, depression, aggression, and other behavior problems. Whether a trait is an asset or a risk factor depends on the environment. When there is a "good fit" between the environment and temperament, the child fairs well. For example, imagine that a child prone to negative emotionality has a harsh, punitive father. This is a bad fit, and the child is likely to develop emotional and behavior problems. If the same child has a warm, but firm, father, the child may become less negative. One way to tell if there is a good or bad fit with a child's temperament is to ask adults who live or work with the child (e.g., parents, teachers) what they see as the most annoying traits in *any* child, and then rate the *target child* on these traits. Those who perceive the child as having more "annoying" traits are less likely to provide a good fit environment for that child. For example, one adult may find exuberantly active children fun, but another finds them annoying; which adult is more likely to provide space and time for physical play? Most aspects of temperament do not lead to problems in children. Even children with "difficult" temperament can develop secure attachment and develop well when there is a good fit to their social environment. Thus, temperament is not a determinant of how your life develops.

Gender Identity

Infants just a few months old can distinguish male faces from female faces. Once they figure out their own gender, they become "detectives" actively trying to figure out what boys do and what girls do. Then, they pay more attention to objects and activities that align with their own gender. For example, boys play more with trucks, and girls play more with dolls. Early gender detective activity generally progresses in the sequence shown in Table 3.2. Despite being gender detectives, young children do not yet have the concept that gender is constant across time and situations. Young preschoolers may say that if a boy puts on a skirt, he is now a girl. *Gender constancy* emerges around ages 3–4 but isn't fully developed until about age 7.

Gender segregation occurs across countries and is driven by the children, not adults. When adults are not in control, gender segregation is more pronounced. When children are in group settings, like childcare, they tend to show stronger gender-typed play (Bennet et al., 2020). As children grow from 2 to 5 years of age, they increasingly resist crossing gender boundaries. They demand activities

Table 3.2 Early Development of Gender Detection

Approximate Age	Development
Newborn	Infants distinguish male and female faces
18 months	Toddlers know which toys are for boys and which are for girls
24 months	Toddlers can label individuals as boys or girls
30 months	Gender segregation begins; toddlers prefer to play with same-gender playmates when there is a choice

for their gender and reject activities for the other gender. Preschoolers even enforce gender boundaries on each other, such as "you can't play with that, it's for boys!" Boys and girls are equally likely to be enforcers (Xiao et al., 2019).

By kindergarten, children are aware of gender stereotypes, like what kinds of jobs are held more by women than men, or that daddy should drive the car, not mommy. Young children are capable of learning stereotypes from off-hand comments, like "boys are better at math." You should be careful what stereotypes you teach in casual conversations. As children go through the preschool years, they become absurdly rigid about stereotypes. A female physician was dismayed when her 4-year-old daughter insisted that girls could not be doctors, yet she lived with proof this wasn't true. This is normal development. By age 10, the physician's daughter will no longer hold such rigid stereotypes.

Racial Identity

Children are aware of race from infancy. At 9 months of age, infants distinguish faces from their own race better than those from other races, and they prefer and pay more attention to same-race faces (Pauker et al., 2016). At 6 years of age, children can accurately sort others based on race. This awareness does not influence behavior in preschoolers. Between ages 2 and 4, children share toys equally with same- and other-race peers and show no preference when choosing a playmate (Anzures et al., 2013). However, by ages 4–5, most children begin to show a preference for playing with children from their own racial group.

Strategies to Foster Social–Emotional Competence in Early Childhood

There are numerous ways to improve the social–emotional competence of young children. Depending on your role (parent, therapist, teacher, social worker, etc.) there may be specific programs or interventions for you to use. The following are some research-based general strategies. However, keep in mind that you need to be aware of the ability, rate of development, and culture of each child. When working with children from a culture other than your own, approach the situation with cultural humility (see Chapter 6).

How Can You Form Secure Attachment-Like Relationships?

Among the most powerful ways you help young children develop social–emotional competence is to support the formation of a secure parent–child attachment. You can also form an attachment-like relationship (e.g., teacher–student, therapist–client) with children you work with that can serve some of the same functions as a secure attachment with parents. You will find it easier to form a trusting relationship with children who already have a secure attachment to their parents. Yet, children with insecure attachment may be those who most need a positive relationship with you.

To form an attachment-like relationship, you should be consistently sensitive, responsive, and accepting toward the child. This pattern of behavior disconfirms an insecure child's belief that adults are hostile, uncaring, or untrustworthy. You can use "banking time" where you spend 5–15 minutes per day giving the child undivided attention and following the child's lead in activities. Study child development (like this book) because professionals with greater knowledge of child development are more sensitive toward children. However, be aware that forming attachment-like relationships takes time. For example, it may take 9 months for a child to attach to a childcare provider. Thus, in your professional capacity, try to stay with the same child as long as possible so that trusting relationships can form.

How Can You Help Young Children Develop Emotion Regulation Skills?

In addition to forming attachment-like relationships, you help children learn emotion regulation in these ways:

1. Create an emotionally safe environment. Express mostly positive emotions. However, it is good to occasionally express negative emotions so that you can model how to cope constructively with anger, sadness, or frustration.
2. Talk about emotions whenever the opportunity arises. Help children label, describe, and understand emotions they see around them. Some books and media (e.g., Sesame Street) are designed to facilitate this. Children who can talk about their own and others' emotions are better able to control their emotions.
3. Create a friendly, prosocial environment. We will discuss how to do this below.
4. Co-regulate young children. Let's see how to do this with infants and toddlers next.

How Can You Co-regulate an Infant?

Research has confirmed five techniques that calm infants: (1) snuggly swaddle them with arms at the side, no head covering, and legs flexed (this is important for hip development); (2) hold them on their side, so their startle reflex is not triggered; (3) shush them – "Sh Sh Sh" – rhythmically and loudly; (4) sway, rock, or jiggle gently while providing head support; and (5) give them something to suck. Infants calm faster even after getting immunizations when medical providers use these techniques.

How Can You Handle Toddlers' Tantrums?

You help children outgrow tantrums by co-regulating them. So, how should you handle a tantrum? Ideally, calm the child *before* it begins. You can reduce the frequency of tantrums by eliminating stress, having predictable routines (children thrive on routines), and anticipating exhaustion and hunger. For example, avoid taking young children on a 4-hour shopping trip or to social gatherings past their bedtimes. Once a child is in the middle of a full-blown tantrum, do nothing (unless the child or others are in danger). Do not try to comfort or reason with the child because it will only prolong the anger. Do not give any attention to the tantrum or give in to the child's demands because this will reinforce tantrums. Do not punish the child, and do not worry about other people judging you. Keep in mind that tantrums are episodes of intense sadness, with peaks of anger. Wait until the peaks of anger abate and mere sadness is left, then cuddle and comfort. Sad children seek comfort.

How Can You Help Young Children Become More Prosocial?

There are several ways to increase children's prosocial behavior. The most important are creating a secure attachment-like relationship and using inductive discipline that is described in Chapter 4. You also increase prosocial behavior when you help children develop emotional competence. Children who read other's emotions well and who can regulate their own emotions have more empathy. Especially, point out their peers' good behavior because children are inspired to imitate others. "Look at how kind Lucy is to help me clean up the toys! Helping others is important."

Praise children when they are prosocial. Children who are praised for prosocial behavior tend to behave more prosocially, particularly if the praise comes from an adult with whom they have a warm relationship. It is more powerful to *praise the child* ("You are a helper") rather than the act ("That was helpful") because praising the child builds the child's identity as someone who is kind and helpful. Children interpret their behavior as "I did that because I am the kind of person who likes to help others," which may lead them to behave prosocially in the future. However, do not give the children tangible rewards (e.g., stickers, treats) for being prosocial. Tangible rewards might increase prosocial behavior in the short-term, but they undermine children's motivation to be prosocial in the long-term. Should they expect to be paid to be good?

Give children opportunities to practice being prosocial toward others. This can include tasks in the family or school. We want prosocial behavior to become a well-worn habit. Above we gave the example that if someone drops an object, you allow children to pick it up, and praise them for being good helpers, rather than stepping in to pick it up yourself. Look for similar ways to build prosocial habits.

How Can You Help Young Children Develop Better Self-Control?

Again, an answer is to build secure attachment-like relationships and use inductive discipline. You will see this answer over and over again in this book because these are powerful tools in promoting all dimensions of social–emotional competence. Children with secure attachment tend to have higher self-control for their age, presumably because their parents respond to them sensitively and help scaffold their self-control development. Children who are disciplined with induction also tend to have higher self-control.

You can change situations to promote self-control. Put temptations out of sight. Reduce distractions or interruptions. Help children divert themselves, such as sing songs while they wait for something. Keep them fed because the brain needs fuel to drive self-control; that is why you have less self-control when you are hungry. Do activities that require high levels of self-control earlier in the day; your self-control wanes as the day goes on. Self-control is like a muscle. It grows with practice, but it can also be fatigued. If you overtax self-control in a situation, without rest or chance to reset, it is more likely to fail. For example, it may not be wise to ask children to sit still for too long without a break. At the same time, they do need practice stretching their capacity a little so that it grows over time.

Chapter Summary

Infants and toddlers communicate with their emotions because they lack language. Emotions like happiness, anger, and interest are present at birth, and more complex social emotions like embarrassment, shame, and guilt develop later, by about 3 years of age. Children learn emotion regulation from their AFs during routine activities such as eating and playing. Securely attached children tend to have better emotion regulation than insecure children. Even children with good emotion regulation may have tantrums because they are common in toddlers from about age 1 to 2.

Infants are prosocial beings; they are kind, empathic, and want to help others. However, the desire to be prosocial declines as toddlers recognize that there is a cost to helping others, like giving up their favorite cookie or blanket. Children tend to be more prosocial if they are securely attached, emotionally competent, praised for prosocial behavior, and if they have practice.

Toddlers are aggressive, and 3-year-olds are the most aggressive of any age group. They will grab, hit, and yell to get what they want; imagine an adult displaying the behaviors of a 3-year-old! Theory of mind is important for the development of social competence because it helps children understand other people's perspectives. Infants and toddlers have little self-control, but it grows rapidly. Development of self-control is crucial for social competence, achievement, and overall well-being. Temperament includes four components: activity level, negative emotionality, behavioral inhibition, and behavioral control. These components are related to social competence and self-control.

Suggested Readings

Brackett, M. (2019). *Permission to feel: The power of emotional intelligence to achieve well-being and success*. Celadon/Macmillan.
Karp, H. (2003). *The happiest baby on the block*. Bantam.

References

Anzures, G., Quinn, P. C., Pascalis, O., Slater, A. M., Tanaka, J. W., & Lee, K. (2013). Developmental origins of the other-race effect. *Current Directions in Psychological Science, 22*(3), 173–178.
Bennet, A., Kuchirko, Y., Halim, M. L., Costanzo, P. R., & Ruble, D. (2020). The influence of center-based care on young children's gender development. *Journal of Applied Developmental Psychology, 69*(4), 101157.
Eisenberg, N., Hofer, C., Sulik, M. J., & Liew, J. (2014). The development of prosocial moral reasoning and a prosocial orientation in young adulthood: Concurrent and longitudinal correlates. *Developmental Psychology, 50*(1), 58–70.
Friedman, N. P., Miyake, A., Robinson, J. L., & Hewitt, J. K. (2011). Developmental trajectories in toddlers' self-restraint predict individual differences in executive functions 14 years later: A behavioral genetic analysis. *Developmental Psychology, 47*(5), 1410–1430.
Hay, D., Hurst, S., Waters, C., & Chadwick, A. (2011). Infants' use of force to defend toys: The origins of instrumental aggression. *Infancy, 16*(5), 471–489.
Heyes, C. (2016). Born pupils? Natural pedagogy and cultural pedagogy. *Perspectives on Psychological Science, 11*(2), 280–295.
Martin, A., & Olson, K. R. (2015). Beyond good and evil: What motivations underlie children's prosocial behavior? *Perspectives on Psychological Science, 10*(2), 159–175.
Pauker, K., Williams, A., & Steele, J. R. (2016). Children's racial categorization in context. *Child Development Perspectives, 10*(1), 33–38.
Romano, E., Babchishin, L., Pagani, L. S., & Kohen, D. (2010). School readiness and later achievement: Replication and extension using a nationwide Canadian survey. *Developmental Psychology, 46*(5), 995–1007.
Saylor, K. E., & Amann, B. (2016). Impulsive aggression as a comorbidity of attention-deficit/hyperactivity disorder in children and adolescents. *Journal of Child and Adolescent Psychopharmacology, 26*(1), 19–25.
Schlam, T. R., Wilson, N. L., Shoda, Y., Mischel, W., & Ayduk, O. (2013). Preschoolers' delay of gratification predicts their body mass 30 years later. *Journal of Pediatrics, 162*(1), 90–93.

Tan, L., Volling, B. L., Gonzalez, R., LaBounty, J., & Rosenberg, L. (2022). Growth in emotion understanding across early childhood: A cohort-sequential model of firstborn children across the transition to siblinghood. *Child Development, 93*(3), e299–e314.

Vlachou, M., Andreou, E., Botsoglou, K., & Didaskalou, E. (2011). Bully/victim problems among preschool children: A review of current research evidence. *Educational Psychology Review, 23*(3), 329–358.

Woodard, K., Zettersten, M., & Pollak, S. D. (2022). The representation of emotion knowledge across development. *Child Development, 93*(3), e237–e250.

Xiao, S. X., Cook, R. E., Martin, C. L., & Nielson, M. G. (2019). Characteristics of preschool gender enforcers and peers who associate with them. *Sex Roles, 81*(11), 671–685.

Chapter 4

Social and Emotional Competence in Middle Childhood (Ages 6–12)

In a 4th grade gifted and talented class, Deepak is unable to manage emotions. While programming small robots, he got frustrated, threw himself on the floor, and started crying. His teacher, who is accustomed to Deepak's outbursts, says "If you need me to help, I will. If you don't want help, then you need to go for a walk with the counselor because you are disturbing the other students." Indeed, the other students have stopped their work to watch Deepak. They look on with some compassion, but no one wants to have Deepak on their team.

Why does Deepak behave like this? Does it matter that classmates reject Deepak? What can you do to help children like Deepak? In this chapter, you will learn the answer to these questions as we discuss social–emotional development in middle childhood.

Middle childhood refers to the period from about age 6 to 12. At this age, in most countries, children start attending "elementary" or "primary" school and begin to take on important responsibilities, such as tending younger siblings or taking care of livestock. To launch our discussion on development of social–emotional competence in middle childhood, we begin this chapter with a discussion of discipline. Discipline and attachment (see Chapter 2) are two dimensions of parenting that powerfully influence children's development.

Discipline

Many people mistakenly think that "discipline" means to punish children. Instead, it refers to attempting to change a child's behavior – getting them to stop doing something unacceptable or get them to start doing something desirable. If you work with children, you will need to redirect or correct their behavior *many times every day*. It is important to discipline children in a way that teaches them good values and acceptable behavior so that they can thrive in their social world. *The goal of discipline should be to teach, not to punish.*

Discipline affects children's emotional competence in at least two ways. First, when adults over-react or harshly punish a child's misbehavior, the child is

DOI: 10.4324/9781003046455-4

overwhelmed by emotions (e.g., shame, remorse, anger). This makes it difficult for children to regulate their own emotions – whether the child is a toddler or a teenager – and can make them dislike the punisher. Second, it is in discipline encounters that children learn empathy and values. It may surprise you, but you are most likely to have learned the values you hold during the times you were disciplined. Let's see how this might happen.

Types of Discipline

Adults discipline children in three basic ways: (1) induction, (2) psychological control, and (3) power assertion. Induction is the most effective form of discipline for helping children develop social–emotional well-being, so let's begin there.

Inductive discipline is where the adult explains the *reason for rules* or *why* a child should not engage in certain behaviors and should engage in other behaviors. A particularly important form is *other-oriented* (sometimes called victim-centered) induction, where you point out how the child's misbehavior affected someone else. For example, "We don't tell our friends that they can't play because it hurts their feelings. Look, he feels sad because you excluded him. How would you feel if others wouldn't let you join the game?" Inductive discipline centers on teaching principles that children can apply to later situations. This is how children learn *self*-control and empathy. In addition, if children misbehave because they don't have specific skills or don't know what is expected of them, induction allows you to teach the missing skill.

Psychological control (sometimes called love-withdrawal) is where the adult controls the child by withdrawing affection, disapproving of the child (rather than the behavior), or trying to make the child feel shame or excessive guilt. Psychological control includes ignoring the child, stating dislike for the child, or asking the child why he or she is so bad. For example, "Why can't you ever do anything right?" While induction appeals to children's reason, psychological control makes children fear they will lose adult affection or approval. Of course, some disapproval of the child's behavior is part of any discipline, but it is the central focus of psychological control.

Power assertion is where the adult controls the child through power or resources they have but the child does not have. It includes: (1) physical acts, like hitting or spanking; (2) taking away objects or privileges; (3) bodily constraining or carrying the child away; or (4) threats to do any of the above. For example, "Clean up your room or else you can't go to your friend's house" is power assertion. When adults use the phrase "or else" (even if it isn't stated, but just implied), they are using power assertion.

Let's take a look at examples. Imagine a child comes home from elementary school with a red card for disrupting the class. The parents might respond in these ways:

- Induction: Frown and sternly say "Your teacher put a lot of effort into planning a lesson, and you made it hard for the other students to learn! How would you feel if you were the teacher? You should apologize tomorrow and not do it again."
- Psychological control: "Why are you always embarrassing me and being so bad? Go to your room; I don't want to see your face again today."
- Power assertion: "I warned you! I'm taking your PlayStation away for 3 months!"

Outcomes of Types of Discipline

When children are consistently disciplined with induction, they learn that they can cope with disapproval and repair mistakes. They learn why a principle is important and are more likely to adopt those principles for themselves. They develop greater self-control because they internalize the adult's values, which helps them obey even when the adult isn't hovering over them. They become more empathic toward others and prosocial, rather than antisocial.

Induction may be the most effective form of discipline *regardless of age of the child.* Even toddlers, who are not yet speaking, are more likely to develop better self-control if you use induction. Imagine a toddler is climbing on the counter. You could simply say "No!" and pull the toddler down. But if you say, "Don't climb up there; you'll fall" and pull the toddler down, the toddler is more likely to be compliant with your next request – although you may have to repeat this many times (discipline is seldom a "once-and-done" event). The toddler may not fully understand your reasoning but does understand being treated with respect and kindness.

In contrast, children who are consistently disciplined with psychological control tend to develop more depression, anxiety, delinquency, academic problems, and misbehavior, and less self-confidence or attachment security (Scharf & Goldner, 2018). Psychological control chips away at the child's sense of worth.

Children who are consistently disciplined with power-assertion tend to become angry and resentful toward adults. They also tend to become aggressive because the adult is modeling how to control others with aggression. Unfortunately, power-assertive discipline often leads to obedience in the short-term, which makes adults think it is working so they keep using it. However, a key lesson is that children disciplined with power assertion tend to become less obedient over the long-term; *it backfires by the time children are teenagers*, and often before then. For example, preschoolers who are spanked tend to misbehave more in elementary school (Laible et al., 2020), and teenagers whose parents yell at them tend to become *more* misbehaving and depressed.

There are other costs to power assertion:

1. Children come to *expect* power assertion and threats *before* they will comply. They learn to ignore mild threats so that you have to use stronger and stronger threats over time.
2. Children may not internalize the values of the adult. They comply only to avoid punishment.
3. It harms the relationship between child and adult, because no one likes someone who threatens them.

Power assertive discipline can vary from mild to abusive. These costs of power assertive discipline occur even for the seemingly mild and widely endorsed form of punishment known as "time out." Young children report that they feel lonely, rejected and scared when they are placed in time out. Power assertion is related to abuse because over half of physical abuse instances started as attempts stop misbehavior using corporal punishment (Gershoff, 2013).

Rewards and Bribes

Some adults wield power over children by using rewards and bribes. For example, "if you behave well, you'll get a treat." Rewards and bribes do influence behavior – in the short-term. In the moment, the child is likely to behave well in order to get the treat. Still, there are costs to this seemingly positive form of power assertion: (1) You need bigger and bigger rewards, (2) children will begin to ask "what do I get if I do that?" (3) it often devolves into punishment such as "you didn't behave, so you don't get the treat," and (4) the biggest cost is that it undermines self-control. How does it do this? Children learn to rely on rewards to direct their behavior instead of internalizing principles for good behavior.

Parenting Styles

Another powerful influence on children is the warmth of their relationships with parents. Four patterns of parenting are described by the combination of warmth and control:

1. **High control/High warmth = Authoritative**. These parents are very high in control meaning that they guide their children, have consistent routines, and expect mature, polite behavior from their children. They use induction and allow negotiation from their children. These parents respect and cooperate with their children when reasonable. In turn, their children tend to become very high in self-control and self-esteem and do well in school. The children's development gets better over time, so that they become flourishing adolescents (Padilla-Walker et al., 2012). See Figure 4.1.

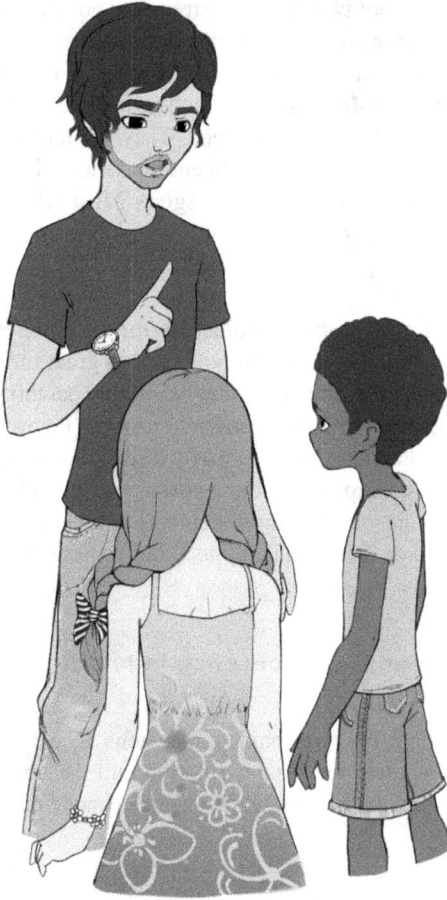

Figure 4.1 Using inductive discipline is a powerful strategy for promoting pro-social behavior and self-control. It is characteristic of authoritative parents.

2. **High control/Low warmth = Authoritarian**. These parents are like a drill sergeant, saying "because I say so!" They use power assertion and do not tolerate negotiation from their children. The children are low-average in self-esteem, average in school, and may (or may not) be compliant while under their parents' thumbs, but they misbehave when turned loose – such as when they move out as young adults.
3. **Low control/Low warmth = Uninvolved** (sometimes called "neglectful"). These parents are not interested in or available to their children. They don't set rules. Their children have low self-control and are delinquent (Clark et al.,

2015). They tend to come from two income extremes – poverty and wealth. Wealthy parents may be too busy to spend time with their children. In addition, some parents may abuse alcohol or drugs which can lead to neglect.

4. **Low control/High warmth = Indulgent** (sometimes called "permissive"). These parents want to be their children's friend. They do not impose rules. Their children tend to have adequate self-esteem but tend to be delinquent and peer-oriented. Few parents fall in this category. Most who are low in control are simply not invested in parenting and fall into the uninvolved category above.

Authoritative parenting is linked to better outcomes for all children, but the difference between authoritative and authoritarian is not as great for Black and Asian children, perhaps because the meaning of authoritarian parenting is interpreted or received differently by children in different groups (Pomerantz et al., 2014; Soenens et al., 2015). Parenting style is partly a reflection of the context the parents live in. Parents who experience the world as unsafe and who find it difficult to earn an adequate income are more likely to be harsh with their children. Parents who are single or lack social support find it more difficult to be authoritative.

Development of Emotional Competence in Middle Childhood

In Chapter 1, you learned that the two major dimensions of emotional competence are the ability to regulate one's own emotion and the ability to read others' emotions. Let's see how both of these dimensions change during middle childhood.

Emotion Regulation – Coping Strategies

Recall from Chapter 1 that you control your emotions by using coping strategies. You learned in Chapter 3 that even infants have some coping strategies. However, children do not use one of the most constructive coping strategies – reappraisal – until around age 7. This is partly because at age 7, children begin to understand that beliefs, rather than the situation, cause emotions. By age 10, emotionally healthy children will have nearly adult-like ability to regulate their own emotions, although they may occasionally break down. How do scientists know this? One way is to use a "disappointing gift" test where scientists give children a baby toy as a gift. Young children get mad or cry in response. By age 8, many children can mask their disappointment with the gift, although it might leak out through biting their lip, touching their face, and glancing at the experimenter. By age 10, most children can hide their disappointment and smile at the scientist. They can regulate their emotions.

In Chapter 1, you learned that coping strategies can be either *problem-* or *emotion-focused*. By age 6–12, children understand that which strategy is best depends on the situation. They believe the best strategy to cope with sadness is to talk to their parents, the best strategy for being taunted is to walk away, and the worst strategy overall is to be aggressive. They can handle many, but not all, emotional situations on their own. Interview Box 4.1 illustrates how two social workers helped youth develop better emotional competence.

Reading Others' Emotions (Affective Perspective-Taking)

Both emotion contagion and social referencing (see Chapter 1) continue to occur in middle childhood and through adulthood. However, children will use social referencing less often with age because fewer situations are ambiguous to older children. During the middle years, children come to understand that: (1) others can fake their emotions, (2) others can have multiple, competing emotions, and (3) others' beliefs can be inferred from their emotions. For example, if someone says they like your new haircut, but then smirk behind your back, a 10-year-old can infer that the other person didn't really like your haircut. And that 10-year-old might also infer that while the other person appears "disapproving" of the new haircut, the person may actually be "jealous." These are sophisticated skills! Children in middle childhood learn to skillfully use more complex emotion words like "jealous" and "disapproving."

Box 4.1   Interview with Two Social Workers

In her interview (Box 1.3), Leslie mentioned that she once worked with a child who tried to stab a classmate with a pencil. Although in middle school, the child had trouble verbalizing emotions, especially when angry or upset. She used her knowledge of social–emotional competence and her knowledge of play/art therapy. She suggested he draw interactions that upset him, and he did. This prompted him to discuss what happened. His drawings helped him uncover what upset him and why he behaved the way he did. He discussed his frustrations and recognized that his behavior was inappropriate. Through Leslie's suggestions, he learned better ways to handle frustrations in the future.

Rita, now a retired social worker and educational administrator who worked with elementary and middle school children for more than 45 years, said that social–emotional competence affected all aspects of her work with children. It affects both interpersonal (meaning "between" people) and intrapersonal (meaning "within" a person) experiences. It helps with relationships and self-awareness. Both Leslie and Rita learned about social–emotional development during their MA social work programs. Rita furthered her knowledge with additional graduate work in educational administration and Leslie completed a clinical internship.

Development of Social Competence in Middle Childhood

Attachment

The attachment *relationship* continues to be important in middle childhood because children still need to feel safe and secure. However, attachment *behaviors* are dramatically different. Older children need less physical contact with attachment figures (AFs) compared to toddlers, although they still like to be in proximity. For example, children may choose to sit near a parent while doing their homework. Older children also no longer have separation distress unless the situation is extreme (e.g., mother is being taken away in an ambulance).

In middle childhood, securely attached children feel comfortable expressing negative feelings toward the AF without fearing abandonment; negative feelings are easily resolved. Secure children tend to do well in school and are well-liked. Compared to insecure children, secure children in middle childhood tend to have greater empathy for others, more harmonious friendships, and greater resistance to negative peer pressure. Adults perceive them as socially competent.

Insecurely attached children may avoid their AF or exclude the AF, such as turning their back on the AF. They may seem to be in control but are actually anxious. If they seek contact with the AF, they are not comforted. They may hide negative emotions to protect themselves from rejection by the AF. They find it difficult to discuss emotions. Alternatively, they may be overly clingy, unable to separate from the AF in age-appropriate situations (e.g., going to school). They may try to control their AF through tantrums, pouting, whining, or acting helpless or babyish. They behave in immature or hyperactive ways. They tend to have lower test scores and grades, perhaps because their anxiety interferes with learning.

Prosocial Behavior

You learned in Chapter 3 that preschoolers who are highly social may be prosocial *and* antisocial. This is no longer the case in middle childhood because older children tend to specialize as either more prosocial ("nice kids") or antisocial ("mean kids") and stay that way. This means that the same child is likely to be consistently above average in prosocial or antisocial behavior through middle childhood and into adulthood.

Children who are more prosocial benefit in important ways. They have higher achievement at school, where they listen, stay on-task, work better with others, and learn more. They are more likely to be calm, happy, well-liked, and have more positive relationships with peers and teachers in the classroom. They are less likely to be negatively affected by risk, trauma, or adversity. They are less likely to be held back a grade or be in special education throughout their schooling. This means prosocial behavior is a protective factor that helps children be resilient. These positive effects of prosocial behavior occur for all children, but especially for impoverished students (Bergin, 2018).

Antisocial Behavior

Overall, children are less aggressive in middle childhood compared to younger ages, but when they are aggressive, they use verbal or social aggression more than physical. Social aggression begins to appear around age 8. They are also less likely to use instrumental aggression, but more likely to use retaliation and bullying. Keep in mind that not all aggression is bullying. Aggression is bullying when there is an imbalance of power in a relationship and the aggressor intends to harm, seeks power, and is not remorseful. Typically, bullying is repeated, although a one-time event can be considered bullying.

As many as 20%–30% of school children may be victimized by bullies in a given year (Irwin et al., 2022). For most children, it does not last, but for some children, it can last for years. Being a victim puts children at risk for problems such as low grades, feeling anxious or angry at school, peer rejection, poor sleep, and low self-esteem.

Above, you learned that at this age, children tend to specialize in either prosocial or antisocial behavior. Most children are not aggressive and about 20% are aggressive when young but taper off. About 15% of children stay aggressive over time. These are more likely to be boys; gender differences get larger with age. Thus, aggressive children you work with are not likely to simply outgrow it (with the exception of preschoolers). Children who continue to be physically aggressive, as well as argumentative and have tantrums past age 8, may be diagnosed with conduct disorder (Table 1.1).

Theory of Mind

Children's ability to read others' minds grows in middle childhood. They become able to make a persuasive argument. For example, "Can we get a dog? I'll take it for a walk every day after school, and it will keep Grandpa company." The child has to read the parents' minds and address objections before they are even made. This is an impressive skill. Children also become better at inferring intent of story characters – "I think he didn't really want to do it, even though he said he did." This allows them to read more sophisticated literature. Children with better theory of mind are liked better because it helps them to see others' perspectives when making a joke or resolving a conflict. They also tend to be more prosocial (Imuta et al., 2016).

Friends and Peers

In middle childhood, children begin to spend more time with friends and peers than with adults. Let's see how this develops.

Friendships

Most (85%) children average 3–8 friends in middle childhood. It is common for friendships to change from one year to the next. Despite shifts in *who* a child is friends with, *whether* a child has friends, and the *quality* of those friendships is stable. This means that a child who has friends one year is still likely to have friends the next year, but they may be different friends. Friendships may be more stable if the friends are quite similar (e.g., same academic achievement level or participate in the same sports).

Children tend to choose friends who are similar to themselves in gender, academic achievement, athleticism, religiosity, ethnicity, aggressiveness, and mental health. Friends tend to "select" others who are similar to them and then "socialize" each other to be even more similar. They do this by teasing, pressuring, reinforcing, and modeling. This is commonly known as "peer pressure." Many think of peer pressure as negative, but this is misguided (Laursen & Veenstra, 2023). *Most peer pressure is positive*, meaning that friends pressure each other to do the right thing.

Friendships are good for children if they are of high quality. They provide enjoyment, comfort, and belonging. Friends talk about emotions with each other, which helps children learn to regulate their own emotions and understand others' emotions. However, low-quality friendships can be a risk factor when "friends" are mean and pressure each other to be antisocial. Children who are insecurely attached to parents tend to be more susceptible to negative peer pressure, whereas securely attached children tend to have high-quality friendships.

Middle childhood is the peak of gender segregation meaning that girls are friends with girls, and boys with boys. By age 10, 95% of friends and cliques are same-gender. Children will actively avoid opposite-sex peers in contexts, such as school, where they have access to multiple peers. This may not occur in a small neighborhood where there isn't a lot of choice in playmates.

Friends also tend to segregate by ethnicity somewhat, but not as markedly as by gender. Prosocial children tend to have more cross-ethnic friendships because others want to be friends with them regardless of ethnicity. The extent of cross-ethnic friendships depends on opportunity. In U.S. schools, White children are more likely to have cross-ethnic friendships compared to Black or Latino students. Children who are a small, ethnic minority in their school tend to stick together with fewer cross-ethnic friendships. Box 4.2 illustrates how social competence plays out in a school lunch room.

Box 4.2   Lunchroom Case Study

A researcher observed fourth graders at lunch in two schools in Los Angeles (Nukaga, 2008). The schools were predominantly Korean and included White, Hispanic, and Black students. She found that children really wanted to sit with friends and would enter the cafeteria together and save seats for each other. Boys and girls almost never sat together, but tables tended to be ethnically mixed. She found that children classified food as wet (e.g., homemade sandwiches, soup, and rice) or dry (e.g., packaged cookies, chips, and seaweed). Dry food was easily shared with others, but wet food was only shared with close friends: "I often watched kids giving their food to their closest friends with chopsticks and forks that they had been using" (p. 360). Kids traded food, but they also gave food as gifts, especially to best friends. Newcomers gave food as bids to become friends. Kids often gave food to peers whom they did not even know. What do the patterns of behavior in these fourth graders show about prosocial behavior, ethnic differences, gender segregation, and peer status?

Peer Status

Friend groups may combine to form "cliques" or social groups from 5 to 40 friends. Children become part of different social groups, such as a classroom, athletic team, church youth group, and so on. Peer status refers to a child's standing in the social group. It is measured by asking children who in the group they like and want to work or play with, and who they dislike most. Based on responses, children within the group are classified in five ways:

1. Average (about 50% of children). These children receive a moderate number of nominations and tend to be average in both prosocial and aggressive behavior.
2. Well-liked (about 15% of children). These children receive many "like" and few "dislike" nominations. Their most stand-out characteristic is *high levels of prosocial behavior*. They have many friends and are social leaders.
3. Rejected (about 15% of children). These children receive few "like" and many "dislike" nominations. Their standout features are *high levels of aggression* or *socially odd behaviors*. The odd behaviors can include extreme

shyness, depression, highly fragile feelings that are easily hurt, crying a lot, or making odd noises. Deepak in the opening vignette is rejected in his class because he has tantrums. Rejected children are actively disliked, not merely ignored.

4. Neglected (about 10% of children). These children receive few of both kinds of nominations. They tend to have few friends.

5. Controversial (about 6% of children). These children receive many "like" *and* "dislike" nominations. Their most stand-out characteristic is being pro-social sometimes and aggressive sometimes, depending on which suits their purpose. They often read others well, strategically using aggression with subtlety. They trigger strong reactions from other children. Even when disliked, they manage to be prominent and have social impact. They may have athletic prowess or be especially good looking (Ettekal & Ladd, 2015).

You can readily identify these groups by second grade. They are fairly stable, meaning that a child who is rejected in second grade is likely to be rejected in high school as well.

Notice that behavior (prosocial or antisocial) is the strongest predictor of a child's peer status. Given that behavior is a function of the child's life experience, the same experiences that lead to antisocial behavior are linked to peer rejection: insecure attachment, harsh power-assertive discipline, a critical father, and marital conflict/divorce. Experiences linked to being well-liked include secure attachment and parents' use of inductive discipline. One caveat is that whether an aggressive child is rejected for being aggressive depends on the norm of the group. For example, boy groups have higher levels of aggression, so boys may be less rejected for being aggressive than girls would be.

Peer status affects well-being. Not surprisingly, well-liked children fare well, while rejected children fare worse. When children are rejected for a year or longer, they tend to experience distress, increased aggression, depression, loneliness, and low self-esteem (although some who are bullies may have inflated self-esteem). They have low academic achievement, perhaps because they give up on challenging tasks and disengage or misbehave in the classroom. They have high levels of cortisol (a stress hormone) while at school and may drop out (Spilt et al., 2014).

Shyness

Shyness is discomfort with social situations. Shyness is common in younger children but tends to abate in middle childhood. In American culture, many adults see shyness as a problem, but in other cultures it is considered a virtue. Be aware of your bias and do not confuse shyness with poor social skills or low self-esteem (which is anxiety about one's self-worth). In Chapter 2, you learned that shyness can be a protective asset; it tends to protect children from aggression and injuries. You do not need to be concerned about shy-sociable children (see Chapter 2), but shy-non-sociable children or extreme shyness beyond fourth grade might warrant intervention. If there is an underlying anxiety disorder, extremely shy children can be rejected by peers. Key factors to watch for are: (1) does the child have friends? Children tend to develop fine as long as they have one good friend. (2) Does the child do things alone that are normal to do alone (e.g., read a book) or do things alone that are normal to do with others (e.g., play with a ball alone on a playground filled with classmates). (3) Does the child appear socially unskilled for their age?

Development of the Self in Middle Childhood

Self-Control

In Chapter 3, you learned what self-control is, and how it increases in young children. You learned about the marshmallow task to measure "delay of gratification." In middle childhood, children can wait longer for their second marshmallow compared to preschoolers, shifting from just seconds to several minutes of waiting. Scientists also measure self-control by asking children to do a task while there are distractions going on (e.g., flashing lights, music playing). Preschoolers have a hard time ignoring the distractions, but by middle childhood, they are more successful.

Children who have high self-control in middle childhood tend to do better in school, earning higher grades and test scores. They pay attention and stay on task in school. They get along with classmates and teachers. Most people think that being "smart" predicts how well you do in school, but having self-control may be more important to school success.

Self-Esteem

Self-esteem is your overall feeling of being a worthy person. Some children have higher self-esteem than others. Self-esteem is fairly stable. Children with low self-esteem are likely to carry that into adulthood.

Where does healthy self-esteem come from? It is partly a reflection of how the important people in our world view us. Secure attachment is the bedrock of self-esteem because it leads children to believe "I am worthy of love" and "others can be trusted to take care of me." Insecure children receive less parental regard, so they have low self-esteem. They may try to earn parents' affection through super achievement such as becoming a workaholic, or they may become overly anxious to please others, clingy, and emotionally "needy." Without realizing it, children seek friends who confirm their self-image. Securely attached children are likely to make friends with people who support positive self-esteem. Insecure children make friends with people who support low self-esteem.

Self-esteem also comes from a self-assessment of "What am I good at?" You can have different feelings about specific areas of competence – I'm not a good writer, I am a good friend; I'm not a good athlete, I am a good problem-solver. High self-esteem comes from being good at something your family or culture values. Preschoolers have unrealistic views of their skills – they are the smartest one in class, or the fastest one on their soccer team. A 4-year-old will say "watch how high I can jump!" and then barely catch air, but after landing will say "aren't I good at jumping!" In middle childhood, children become more realistic and accurate at self-assessment. This is because they become more competent at comparing their own skills with their peers. Sadly, this means that on average, children's self-assessment of ability tends to go down in middle childhood (Scherrer & Preckel, 2018). Perceptions of competence diminish steadily from first grade to high-school graduation, bottoms out, but then starts to rise again.

Personality

In Chapter 3, you learned about temperament, which is the foundation of personality. Research shows that some aspects of personality have a genetic basis, but most of your personality is not genetic and is shaped by your social experience, particularly attachment and quality of parenting. Experiences shape our personality traits.

Traits

There are many ways you could describe personality, but research finds that just five overarching factors known as the Big Five accounts for much of personality.

1. **Openness to experience**. Creative, curious, enjoy exploring new situations, express themselves well, and get lost in thought and wrapped up in projects.
2. **Conscientiousness**. Neat, orderly, reliable, get things done, do not give up easily, set high standards for themselves, and think before acting. (Related to "effortful control" temperament.)
3. **Extraversion**. Energetic, talkative, sensation seeking, and full of life. They react quickly and show emotions openly. (Related to "behavioral inhibition" and "activity" temperament.)
4. **Agreeableness**. Prosocial, thoughtful of others, warm, kind, helpful, and cooperative.
5. **Neuroticism**. Anxious, worry excessively, go to pieces or get sick under stress, and feel hurt easily. (Related to "negative emotionality" temperament).

The five factors are known by the acronym OCEAN. These personality traits predict important outcomes, even more than intelligence or family income. High conscientiousness, high agreeableness (i.e., prosocial), and low neuroticism predict social–emotional well-being and school success.

Stability

There are two general age trends in personality in middle childhood. Activity level increases from birth through 7–9 years of age when it peaks, and then decreases. This is why second graders seem like they never sit still! Behavioral inhibition – or shyness –is common in young children, but most will overcome it by about fourth grade.

Despite these general age trends, an individual's personality relative to others their same age becomes fairly stable by middle childhood (Bleidorn et al., 2022). Personality is more stable if a trait is intense and if the social environment supports the trait. For example, intensely shy children are more likely to stay that way. For a social environment example, anxious, hovering parents can make their child more shy. However, personality can change even into old age. This is one of the goals of psychotherapy (see Chapter 11).

Culture

Researchers have found the Big Five traits describe personality across various countries. However, the same personality trait may have different value and meaning depending on the culture. For example, shyness is more valued in China than in the USA, but agreeableness and conscientious are highly valued in both countries.

Identity

Gender Identity

Middle childhood is the age of *greatest gender segregation*. At this age, children will punish peers who cross gender boundaries, such as boys playing with girls, or "girl" toys. When there is little choice of playmates, such as at home, boys and girls will play together. Boys who cross gender boundaries tend to get criticized more by their peers than girls who cross boundaries. By the end of elementary school, children begin to be less rigid in their interests and stereotypes, but they also grow in understanding that males disproportionately get more power and respect than females.

Gender identity can be thought of simply as what gender you acknowledge in yourself. Or, it can be thought of as a complex array of your feelings about your gender – such as whether you feel typical of or content with your gender, pressured to conform to your gender, and proud of your gender. Some children may be gender-variant at this age, which means they do not conform to traditional gender identities associated with their sex (i.e., biology). Transgender children may insist they are the opposite sex as early as preschool (Olson et al., 2015). Transgender children may "socially transition," meaning they adopt the dress, behavior, and activities of their preferred gender. The gender identity of young children may change by adolescence (Hässler et al., 2021). Currently, there is too little rigorous research on how gender variance develops or how it is experienced by children to make definitive statements.

Ethnic and Racial Identity

Race and ethnicity can be distinguished, but they overlap. Ethnicity refers to a group of people who share culture, language, and ancestry. The largest ethnic groups in the USA are White, non-Hispanic (60%), Hispanic (19%), Black (14%), and Asian (6%). Increasingly, individuals have mixed ethnicities, like former President Barak Obama. They may feel pressure to choose one identity, but many have a flexible identity and function well in multiple groups.

Similar to gender identity, racial identity can be thought of as simply what ethnicity you acknowledge, or it also can be thought of as a complex array of your feelings about your ethnicity. Members of the same ethnic group can have different ethnic identity, with some feeling their ethnic identity is core to who they are, but others do not have such feelings. Those who have a positive ethnic identity are proud of their group and derive strength from it. Compared to children who lack a positive ethnic identity, children with positive ethnic identity have higher self-esteem, are happier, less depressed or anxious, and less likely to use drugs. The specific ethnic group they identify with is not as strong a predictor as how they feel about their group (Rogers et al., 2015).

Children become aware of gender stereotypes by age 5. They become aware of racial stereotypes by age 10 (e.g., *Asians are good at math*) and also that people may not like others just because of their race. They also become aware that their own group could be stigmatized or less-valued in the larger community, but do not have as great an understanding as they will develop during adolescence. It is a natural impulse to notice race and categorize people (babies do this in the first months of life), but it is important to guard against treating others with less respect or dignity. Most U.S. Black children have experienced disrespectful treatment before adolescence. This can undermine their emotional well-being, such as reduce motivation in school, increase depression, lower self-esteem, raise anxiety, and even increase illness.

Discrimination refers to seeing out-groups in negatively stereotyped ways and feeling they are "lesser" than your in-group. Discrimination is socially and legally unacceptable. Fortunately, it appears to be declining overall, despite disturbing outbreaks. Over the last 2 decades, U.S. citizens report less bias based on race, sexuality, and skin tone (Charlesworth & Banaji, 2022).

Strategies to Foster Social–Emotional Competence in Middle Childhood

In Chapter 3, you learned that among the most powerful ways to help children develop social–emotional competence is to form secure attachment-like relationships and use inductive discipline. This pertains to middle childhood as well. When adults use inductive (rather than power assertive) discipline, children learn values and self-control. They also learn empathy and prosocial behavior. This is because other-oriented induction (see above) involves asking children "how would you feel if ...." and suggesting how to make amends to restore the relationship and the others' well-being if they have misbehaved. This trains children to consider others' perspectives and needs before they act. Recall that children with authoritative parents are more likely to be prosocial. Authoritative parents use inductive discipline and hold children to a high standard of behavior, while also being warm. You can do the same in any role you have while working with children.

To promote social–emotional competence in middle childhood you will use some of the same strategies you learned in Chapter 3. That is: (1) form attachment-like relationships, (2) talk about emotions, (3) express an array of emotions, but create a primarily emotionally positive environment, and (4) praise and value prosocial behavior, giving children opportunity to be helpful and kind to others. In addition, you can use the following strategies.

How Can You Coach Children's Coping Strategies?

Unlike preschoolers, in middle childhood, you should no longer need to "co-regulate" a typical child's emotions. However, most children will need your help to constructively cope with a strong emotion. To coach coping strategies, refer back to the coping strategies in Box 1.1. Should the child take a deep breath, get a drink of water, apologize, run around the block, or reappraise? Consult the child, because at this age they are old enough to discuss constructive strategies. Children whose adults coach them in *reappraisal* and other constructive strategies will learn to control their emotions and cope with stress better. They also develop better health, impulse control, attention, and social competence.

How Can You Help Children Who Are Rejected?

Although peer status is stable, change is possible. Just moving rejected children to a new group will not work. It often takes less than an hour for rejected children to be disliked in the new group. Instead, focus on doing all the things discussed above – particularly building their prosocial behavior and helping them regulate their negative emotions. Another effective approach is to point out what you admire in the child to the other children. If appropriate, give them an opportunity to show off their skills, or pair them with a high-status prosocial peer. This will change the child's peer status as other children come to appreciate the child's strengths, not just the annoying behavior.

How Can You Help Shy Children?

You can help shy children adapt to social situations by giving them control and letting them pace their approach to a new situation. Avoid pushing them into a group, being intrusive, or overly critical. At the same time, avoid hovering and communicating your anxiety about their anxiety. This can increase children's shyness. If you think they might be uncomfortable in a new group, you can keep them with friends (e.g., when starting a new class). Give them repeated, gradual exposure to a new situation. Try to adjust the environment to fit with what makes the child comfortable as the child warms up to the situation.

How Can You Help a Child Have Healthy Self-Esteem?

Simply telling a child "you're great" or asking them to focus on themselves does little to build healthy self-esteem. Instead, do the hard work of looking at yourself. Are you building attachment-like relationships? Are you using induction? Recall that power assertive and psychological control undermine self-esteem; induction builds self-esteem. Do you treat the child with respect? Do you make it clear that you like the child? Or, do you belittle, criticize, or yell at the child? It is feeling worthy of love by those in our social world that leads to healthy self-esteem. In addition, teach the child skills that are valued in the child's community.

How Can You Help Children Develop a Healthy Ethnic/ Racial Identity?

You can promote healthy self-identity without promoting out-group bias. Build children's empathy, theory of mind, and prosocial behavior so that they learn to treat out-group members with dignity. Appreciate the identity of the children you work with. Children who are part of stigmatized groups can fare well if their adults, while pointing out the reality of discrimination, suggest how to cope with their feelings, point out successful members of their group, and teach pride in their ethnic heritage. Mere contact with out-group members does not necessarily reduce prejudice, but cooperating toward shared goals can.

One strategy that does not work is claiming color-blindness. Some people find this surprising because they mistakenly think that ignoring differences and treating everyone the same will make race no longer matter. Research shows that people notice race, which influences perceptions and behaviors. Pretending to ignore race can leave in place attitudes and policies that disadvantage some groups. Ironically, White individuals who appear to ignore race are viewed as *more* prejudiced by African Americans than Whites who do talk about race (Yi et al., 2023).

Chapter Summary

In addition to attachment, discipline is foundational to developing social–emotional competence. The goal of discipline is to teach, not to punish. It is to help children internalize self-control. Inductive discipline emphasizes explaining why behavior needs to change, and is the most effective long-term approach. Psychological control and power assertion have negative consequences. The most effective parenting style is authoritative in which parents are warm but also provide strong guidance and high expectations for children through inductive discipline.

Socially competent children in middle childhood tend to be high in theory of mind skills and prosocial behavior and low in antisocial behavior. Middle childhood is the peak of gender segregation; children also segregate by ethnic/racial group, but less than by gender. Peer status refers to a child's standing in the social group. Well-liked children fare well, while rejected children fare worse. Self-control and healthy self-esteem enhance children's well-being. Personality traits tend to be fairly stable by middle childhood. High conscientiousness, high agreeableness (i.e., prosocial), and low neuroticism predict social–emotional well-being and school success. Gender and ethnic/racial identity are important aspects of the self.

Suggested Readings

Bergin, C. (2018). *Designing a prosocial classroom: Fostering collaboration in students from pre-K-12 with the curriculum you already use*. Norton.

Imuta, K., Henry, J. D., Slaughter, V., Selcuk, B., & Ruffman, T. (2016). Theory of mind and prosocial behavior in childhood: A meta-analytic review. *Developmental Psychology, 52*(8), 1192–1205.

Simmons, R. (2011). *Odd girl out: The hidden culture of aggression in girls*. Revised edition. Mariner Books.

References

Bergin, C. (2018). *Designing a prosocial classroom: Fostering collaboration in students from pre-K-12 with the curriculum you already use*. Norton.

Bleidorn, W., Schwaba, T., Zheng, A., Hopwood, C. J., Sosa, S. S., Roberts, B. W., & Briley, D. A. (2022). Personality stability and change: A meta-analysis of longitudinal studies. *Psychological Bulletin, 148*(7–8), 588–619.

Charlesworth, T. E. S., & Banaji, M. R. (2022). Patterns of implicit and explicit attitudes: I. Long-term change and stability from 2007 to 2016. *Psychological Science, 33*(9), 1347–1371.

Clark, T. T., Yang, C., McClernon, F. J., & Fuemmeler, B. F. (2015). Racial differences in parenting style typologies and heavy episodic drinking trajectories. *Health Psychology, 34*(7), 697–708. https://doi.org/10.1037/hea0000150

Ettekal, I., & Ladd, G. W. (2015). Developmental pathways from childhood aggression–disruptiveness, chronic peer rejection, and deviant friendships to early adolescent rule breaking. *Child Development, 86*(2), 614–631.

Gershoff, E. T. (2013). Spanking and child development: We know enough now to stop hitting our children. *Child Development Perspectives, 7*(3), 133–137.

Hässler, T., Glazier, J. J., & Olson, K. R. (2022). Consistency of gender identity and preferences across time: An exploration among cisgender and transgender children. *Developmental Psychology, 58*(11), 2184–2196.

Imuta, K., Henry, J. D., Slaughter, V., Selcuk, B., & Ruffman, T. (2016). Theory of mind and prosocial behavior in childhood: A meta-analytic review. *Developmental Psychology, 52*(8), 1192–1205. https://doi.org/10.1037/dev0000140

Irwin, V., Wang, K., Cui, J., & Thompson, A. (2022). *Report on Indicators of School Crime and Safety: 2021* (NCES 2022-092/NCJ 304625).

Laible, D., Davis, A., Karahuta, E., & Van Norden, C. (2020). Does corporal punishment erode the quality of the mother–child interaction in early childhood? *Social Development, 29*(3), 674–688.

Laursen, B., & Veenstra, R. (2023). In defense of peer influence: The unheralded benefits of conformity. *Child Development Perspectives, 17*(1), 74–80.

Nukaga, M. (2008). The underlife of kids' school lunchtime: Negotiating ethnic boundaries and identity in food exchange. *Journal of Contemporary Ethnography, 37*(3), 342–380.

Olson, K. R., Key, A. C., & Eaton, N. R. (2015). Gender cognition in transgender children. *Psychological Science, 26*(4), 467–474.

Padilla-Walker, L. M., Carlo, G., Christensen, K. J., & Yorgason, J. B. (2012). Bidirectional relations between authoritative parenting and adolescents' prosocial behaviors. *Journal of Research on Adolescence, 22*(3), 400–408. https://doi.org/10.1111/j.1532-7795.2012.00807.x

Pomerantz, E. M., Ng, F. F.-Y., Cheung, C. S.-S., & Qu, Y. (2014). Raising happy children who succeed in school: Lessons from China and the United States. *Child Development Perspectives, 8*(2), 71–76.

Rogers, L. O., Scott, M. A., & Way, N. (2015). Racial and gender identity among Black adolescent males: An intersectionality perspective. *Child Development, 86*(2), 407–424.

Scharf, M., & Goldner, L. (2018). "If you really love me, you will do/be…": Parental psychological control and its implications for children's adjustment. *Developmental Review, 49*, 16–30. https://doi.org/10.1016/j.dr.2018.07.002

Scherrer, V., & Preckel, F. (2018). Development of motivational variables and self-esteem during the school career: A meta-analysis of longitudinal studies. *Review of Educational Research, 89*(2), 211–258. https://doi.org/10.3102/0034654318819127

Soenens, B., Vansteenkiste, M., & Van Petegem, S. (2015). Let us not throw out the baby with the bathwater: Applying the principle of universalism without uniformity to autonomy-supportive and controlling parenting. *Child Development Perspectives*, *9*(1), 44–49. https://doi.org/10.1111/cdep.12103

Spilt, J. L., van Lier, P. A. C., Leflot, G., Onghena, P., & Colpin, H. (2014). Children's social self-concept and internalizing problems: The influence of peers and teachers. *Child Development, 85*(3), 1248–1256.

Yi, J., Neville, H. A., Todd, N. R., & Mekawi, Y. (2023). Ignoring race and denying racism: A meta-analysis of the associations between colorblind racial ideology, anti-Blackness, and other variables antithetical to racial justice. *Journal of Counseling Psychology, 70*(3), 258–275.

Chapter 5

Social and Emotional Competence in Adolescence (Ages 13–19)

In high school, a math teacher told Nicole, "You're good at this; you should consider majoring in math in college." Nicole did not think of herself as competent in math, but this single comment made her think about math as a career. She ended up getting a master's degree in mathematics.

In contrast, Mitch's identity in math was undermined by a teacher in middle school who gave him a failing grade. This made him believe he was bad at math. He carried this identity with him for several years. Eventually he became a graduate student in psychology. Even when fellow students asked Mitch for help with their statistics class, which requires understanding of math, he still didn't think he was good at math. It wasn't until a professor told Mitch that he was good at math and pointed out that Mitch helped other PhD students that Mitch developed an identity as a person who is good at mathematics.

What influenced Nicole's and Mitch's math identity? How might their identity influence their social–emotional development? In this chapter, you will learn the answers to these and other questions about adolescence.

Adolescence refers to the period from ages 13 through 19 and is referred to as the "teens." For this reason, adolescents are commonly called "teenagers." Sometimes, this period is divided into early (about 11–13), middle (14–16), and late (17–19) adolescence. These ages somewhat correspond to divisions in schools (middle school, junior high, and high school). Adolescence brings significant changes in size and puberty development. Girls are usually done growing, but boys can continue growing through the early 20s (typically ending when they are able to grow a beard). Adolescence also brings additional cognitive capacities (e.g., processing speed, working memory size) that influence the social–emotional development we will discuss in this chapter.

Development of Emotional Competence in Adolescence

Adolescence has been characterized as a period of *storm and stress* with risk-taking, conflict, and difficulties. However, research suggests "storm and stress"

DOI: 10.4324/9781003046455-5

is a myth. Most adolescents are confident, have caring connections with parents and others, focus on making a contribution, and work hard toward goals. The storm and stress myth is dangerous because it leads adults to think that adolescents who actually need mental health support are "just being a normal teenager," so adults do not get them help they need. If an adolescent is chronically unhappy or moody, adults should address the child's needs rather than assume it is just "a normal phase" or simply the result of "raging hormones."

Emotion Regulation

In Chapter 4, you learned that adult-like emotion regulation is in place by about age 10 in typically developing children. However, there is some improvement in adolescence. Teens are more likely than younger children to use constructive coping strategies, particularly *reappraisal,* to regulate their emotions, and they become better at switching between strategies (Silvers, 2022). Thus, you might expect that most adolescents report being happy most of the time. Research has confirmed this. However, adolescents do experience more *boredom* and *loneliness*, and especially *sleepiness*, compared to their parents or younger children. They also are more vulnerable to *social evaluation* emotions, such as feeling *embarrassment,* if they think someone is looking at them. Furthermore, they report feeling more daily *stress* over relationships with friends or parents, romances, and pressure to do well in school.

Where does the storm and stress myth come from? Not all adolescents have emotion regulation skills. In Chapter 1, you learned that the prevalence of depression increases, peaking around 15–17 years, and then decreases. Mental health issues resulting from poor emotion regulation begin, or worsen, during adolescence (Silvers, 2022). Some adolescents are frequently angry, anxious, or sad. This could be due to:

- Sleep deprivation, which affects emotion regulation. Sleep deprivation is an epidemic among adolescents (see discussion below).
- A pile-up of negative events such as a move, a new school, or parents' divorce.
- Insecure attachment, which undermines emotion regulation (see Chapter 2). Insecure adolescents are not able to discuss hot topics without anger or to take on difficult challenges; they tend to fall apart when distressed.
- Parents' use of power assertive discipline (see Chapter 4), which becomes less tolerated by children as they grow into adolescents.

Poor quality of parenting is a primary cause of emotion dysregulation, such as depression, anxiety, and externalizing disorders (Silvers, 2022). The process begins in the first years of life, when parenting quality shapes parts of the brain involved in emotion regulation, which leads to general irritability many years later in adolescence. General irritability is thought to underly emotional disorders.

Where else does the storm and stress myth come from? Adolescents tend to have anxiety about being rejected or ridiculed by peers. They fear social exclusion. It is common for them to think others are staring at and judging them, making them feel self-conscious, when in reality the others are looking at something else (Smith, 2020).

While hypersensitivity to social evaluation is normal, some adolescents develop serious *social anxiety*. These youth expect to be viewed negatively by others. This negative bias (review social cognition bias in Chapter 2) leads to interpreting ambiguous events as negative (like someone who *might* be talking about them), they stew on what *might* be happening (the person talking about them). They conclude that they lack social skills, so they try to escape social situations. If they actively avoid others, they may be rejected, isolated, and victimized. Avoidance diminishes their ability to have friends, so they have less opportunity to develop social skills. You can see how this creates a negative spiral. Interview Box 5.1 illustrates how one social worker helped youth caught in negative spirals.

Teens may be more vulnerable to social anxiety because they are constructing their identity which makes them insecure about themselves. One cautionary note is not to confuse *socially anxious* youth with youth who are *content* to be alone, doing things by themselves (i.e., shy-sociable youth). Ironically, more girls than boys have social anxiety even though girls may develop theory of mind a little faster than boys.

How can you tell if an adolescent is emotionally healthy? They tend to have *more positive than negative emotions*, but some of both. Recall from Chapter 1 that both positive and negative emotions are adaptive. Guilt is a negative emotion that prevents us from harming others. Outrage motivates us to right a wrong. Shame motivates us to conform to the expectations of our social group. Fear keeps us safe. Although it may seem strange at first, you should not protect youth from all negative emotions. Yet, if negative emotions are intense and chronic, they can have lasting harm. So, how do you reconcile this dilemma? You help youth develop constructive coping strategies as they experience negative emotions in reasonable doses so that they learn to regulate their emotions. This helps them grow into adults who are able to channel negative emotions for good causes and can continue to be productive and caring, despite frustration, sadness, or anger.

Box 5.1   Interview with a Social Worker

As a social worker, Tom worked more than 40 years with children, mostly with adolescents. Tom's cases included children with severe emotional and behavioral issues. His goals for their social–emotional competence was the ability to regulate one's own emotions and behaviors, interact with others, solve problems, and communicate effectively. He believes having competence in these areas enriches self-esteem and self-confidence. Tom used play and talk therapy, mentoring, and coordination with other adults to help his young clients. He tried to inspire youth with the goal of social–emotional competence. This goal was complicated because the youth often lived in maladaptive homes. He also had to develop cultural competence to understand the needs of children from different cultural backgrounds.

Reading Others' Emotions (Affective Perspective-Taking)

Adolescents continue to use emotional contagion and social referencing to read others' emotions. They also grow in their understanding that emotions can co-occur, such as someone being sad and afraid at the same time. You might think that this would make adolescents more empathic than younger children. However, research does *not* support this. In fact, some studies find a *decrease* in empathy in adolescence. Teens can be self-centered and choose not to help because they understand the cost of helping better than younger children. On the other hand, as youth come to know about the world, they are able to empathize with suffering across the globe as they imagine the feelings of people in distant places. You will find some youth become passionate about faraway humanitarian causes.

Adolescents who are compassionate toward others are more likely to be prosocial and non-aggressive (Bianchi et al., 2020). However, compassionate teens also need emotion regulation because compassion can overwhelm them with distress. Emotion regulation helps them manage the compassion so that they can be helpful. How do some youth become more compassionate? They are likely to have compassionate mothers who use other-oriented induction, which teaches them to pay attention to how their behavior affects others (Bussey et al., 2015).

Development of Social Competence in Adolescence

Socially competent teens continue to be securely attached to their parents, are more prosocial than antisocial, read other people well, and get along with peers.

Attachment

Attachment behaviors change with age – a 15-year-old no longer cries when Mom leaves to get groceries like a 2-year-old does – but the need to feel secure attachment continues to be critical in adolescence. This may not be obvious to you because teens sometimes avoid their parents, which makes them seem like they don't care about attachment figures (AFs). They may meet friends away from home or not tell their parents about events at school. This active avoidance may last a year or two, before teens mature enough to seek out their parents again. Do not assume age-appropriate striving for independence means teens are not attached to their parents. Secure teens become independent because they know their parents are "always there for them" despite their avoidance behaviors. Secure teens still touch base with parents. For example, they may hang out in the kitchen for a few minutes while parents make dinner before disappearing to their own space.

Some people mistakenly think that teens shift attachment from parents to peers. This is not the case for secure teens; parents (typically mothers) remain the primary AF. Peers may become secondary AFs. However, teens with insecure attachment to parents may become attached to a best friend or a romantic partner. Teens innately need attachment and will seek it elsewhere if parents are not secure AFs. Teens with insecure attachment to parents can fare well if a substitute figure (e.g., coach, youth group leader, grandparent) provides secure attachment.

One way security of attachment is measured in adolescence is by asking a parent and teen to discuss an emotionally "hot" topic, like curfews, grades, or money. They are assessed for whether they express negative emotions freely, listen sensitively and respectfully to each other, resolve anger constructively, and come to mutual solutions with the relationship intact. Some insecure teens avoid discussing hot topics, but when such discussions erupt they are very hostile. Other insecure teens are preoccupied and anxious about their parent, have excessive concern about where the parent is, and have trouble separating from the parent, such as clinging to the parent while shopping.

Attachment is the foundation for both emotional and social competence as well as for personality and healthy self-esteem in adolescence. Youth with secure attachment have better peer relationships. Remember that attachment serves two purposes: it makes youth feel safe and provides a secure base from which to explore the world. Thus, it is not surprising that securely attached teens are more likely to be mentally healthy and to feel liberated to take on challenging tasks. In contrast, insecurely attached teens are more likely to have internalizing (e.g., anxiety and depression) and externalizing (e.g., aggression) disorders and conflicted relationships with teachers.

Prosocial Behavior

Adolescents are more skilled at prosocial behavior compared to younger children. They can be of genuine help to others such as joking them out of sadness, trying to help them solve a problem, helping with schoolwork, and brokering disagreements between friends (Bergin, 2018). They even engage in prosocial behavior online, such as cheering someone up in a chat room. They also desire to contribute to the world in a meaningful way as their social awareness expands beyond their community.

Notwithstanding this greater skill level, adolescents are *not more frequently* prosocial compared to younger children. The rate of prosocial behavior increases to the end of elementary school, takes a dip in middle school with a low point in mid-adolescence (about 10th or 11th grade), then increases again starting in late adolescence (Bergin, 2018; Rimm-Kaufman et al., 2024).

Given how much effort adults (e.g., parents, teachers, pastors) put into teaching children to be kind, and the fact that babies come into the world prewired to be prosocial (see Chapter 3), why aren't adolescents prosocial superstars compared to younger children? There are at least three answers:

1. They become more aware of the costs of prosocial behavior and learn to protect their self-interests better. A focus on "what's in it for me?" may *increase* among adolescents.
2. They may become better at regulating their emotions, so that they do not impulsively respond to others' distress. Thus, prosocial behavior becomes a controlled choice rather than an impulse.
3. They have antisocial and selfish models in their lives and in the media who may suppress their prosocial tendencies. Teens who watch TV or play videogames that are violent and aggressive become more aggressive. Fortunately, teens who watch prosocial TV shows and play prosocial videogames (which are admittedly few) become more prosocial over time (Coyne et al., 2018).

Adolescents who continue to be prosocial benefit in important ways. They tend to have higher grades and test scores. For example, students who are more prosocial in sixth–seventh grade have higher achievement in 12th grade (Curlee et al., 2019). They tend to be happier and less depressed, partly because being kind to others leads to good feelings about yourself, reduces your feelings of stress, helps you maintain a state of calm, and leads to others liking you better. Research supports an old adage that the best cure for loneliness or sadness is serving others.

Antisocial Behavior

Aggression steadily declines from preschool to old age, with the exception of a temporary spike in middle school, particularly in bullying. Bullies are not tolerated much by either younger or older youth, but some bullies can have a type of status in middle school. They may be jocks or seem "cool" because they act and dress older than their age.

The presence of bullies means there are also victims. About 20% of adolescents report being bullied at school (most commonly in the classroom and hallway), 15% report being cyberbullied online, and 6% report being called hate-related names (i.e., verbal aggression). The most common focus of hate speech is race/ethnicity, followed by sexual orientation, gender, religion, and disability (Musu et al., 2019). Targets of racial/ethnic hate-speech at school are fairly evenly divided among Asian, Black, Latino, and White students.

Despite the brief spike in bullying in middle school, keep in mind that most youth are not aggressive and seldom get into trouble. Antisocial behavior is "neither inevitable nor typical" (Gutman et al., 2017, p. 112), again dispelling the myth of adolescence being a time of storm and stress. Some (up to 15%) low-aggressive youth may have a *brief* episode of antisocial behavior in adolescence. This pattern is called *adolescent-onset*. They may engage in some delinquency, increasing from age 12 to about age 15, then decreasing to the end of high school. Which youth have this pattern? It is usually those who have a significant increase in life stress during adolescence, lack parental monitoring, and socialize with delinquent peers. This temporary antisocial behavior does not generally portend long-term problems.

Another group (about 5%–15%) have *childhood-onset* antisocial behavior. This means it begins early and persists. This pattern *does* predict long-term problems. For this group, there may be an increase in aggression around age 15, which then decreases as they enter adulthood. Crimes are most perpetrated in the late teens and young adulthood. Half of criminals commit their first offense between ages 14 and 17.

Aggression can be a problem for adolescents. In Chapter 4, you learned that aggressive children have lower academic achievement. This effect is even stronger in high school compared to elementary school. In high school, aggression can lead to social rejection and dropping out. Aggressive youth may select friends who are also aggressive. They form cliques of antisocial friends as early as age 10, who then socialize each other into antisocial behavior in their teens. You can help children get off this trajectory by building their prosocial behavior.

Theory of Mind

In Chapter 3, you learned that theory of mind – or the ability to understand others' beliefs, intentions, desires, and viewpoint – grows dramatically in early childhood. There is another dramatic surge in adolescence as brain regions involved in people-reading mature. This development makes irony, sarcasm, humor, negotiation, lying, and persuasion possible. For example, if someone says, "I see you got dressed up for the party," when another person shows up looking like they just rolled out of bed, adolescents know the statement meant the opposite of what was said. Younger children do not get sarcastic humor.

This doesn't mean adolescents are perfect at reading other people. One way that theory of mind is measured in adolescents is to show them a picture of a house. Then, the picture is covered so that just one corner shows. Adolescents are then asked, "What would a new person think this was a picture of?" Most will say the new person would think it was a picture of a house, although that is not likely. They assume that others know what they know. Even adults have this bias. Indeed, theory of mind continues to develop into old age.

Some youth, including those with autism, may struggle with theory of mind. This is especially true in complex situations, such as when people don't express the emotion you would expect them to in the situation (Jankowski & Pfeifer, 2021). Some teens who have high levels of empathic concern for others, but poor theory of mind, can develop social anxiety (discussed above). This is because the empathy overwhelms them without understanding others' perspectives or having enough self-regulation to manage their empathy. They focus on their own feelings and are less able to perceive others accurately.

Peer Status

In Chapter 4, you learned that children can be categorized as well-liked, rejected, neglected, or controversial. Similar to younger children, adolescents who are well-liked or average tend to fare better in most peer contexts. Youth who are rejected continue to do poorly in high school, just as they did at younger ages. An interesting phenomenon occurs in adolescence where some youth who are not actually well-liked, and are somewhat antisocial, gain high social status because they are pseudo-mature and seem to act old for their age; for example, they might date or drink earlier than age mates. They are called *perceived popular* to distinguish them from those who are well-liked and pro-social. The social clout of *perceived popular* youth doesn't last long. By young adulthood they are more likely than other youth to use alcohol and other drugs, commit crimes, have relationship problems, and become parents early (e.g., Cole et al., 2024).

Recall from Chapter 4 that most peer pressure is actually positive, rather than negative. Adolescents who are securely attached and have authoritative parents are more likely to give and receive positive peer pressure. Their parents tend to: (1) use inductive discipline, (2) monitor their children's peer interactions, but not directly intervene or over-manage situations, and (3) coach social skills when their children lack social skills or need to be directed away from deviant peers. Such parents might ask "how is X a good friend?" thus revealing that X is not a good friend, and then discuss what makes a good friend. In contrast, parents who are overly protective, discourage independence, or use psychological control discipline (instead of induction) tend to have socially anxious adolescents who are susceptible to negative peer pressure.

Friendships

Adolescents spend more time with friends compared to younger children. It is a common myth that friends replace parents in importance during adolescence. While teens talk about significant issues with their friends, this does not mean that friends replace parents. Teens report talking as much with and feeling greater support from their parents. Thus, friends are an *addition* to teens' social support networks. Youth are more likely to have high-quality friendships if they are prosocial, have secure parent–child attachments, and have good theory of mind skills.

Most youth (80%–90%) have reciprocal friends – that means each nominates the other as a friend – with 2–4 close friends. Friendships and cliques are more stable the older children get, but even in adolescence, best friends and cliques can change from year to year. When friends share similar attributes and interests (e.g., extracurricular activities such as sports, arts, youth groups, and clubs), their friendships tend to be more stable. Similarity among friends in attractiveness, academic achievement, and aggression are stronger for adolescents compared to younger children. Adolescents will often join activities or classes that their friends are in, which then forges additional friendships. Selection of friends based on shared activities occurs in younger children but is stronger in high school.

The extreme gender segregation of middle childhood gives way to more mixed-gender cliques in high school. Adolescents report feeling more confidence when interacting with the opposite gender compared to middle childhood. However, youth who spend more time with other-sex peers in unsupervised settings tend to develop behavior problems, have lower school achievement, and greater depression, so supervision is important (Lam et al., 2014). This crossing of gender boundaries can lead to early romance in adolescence (see Figure 5.1).

Early Romance

"Romance" goes beyond friendship, is more intense, affectionate, and may or may not involve intimacy. Showing interest in the opposite sex while adolescents' social skills are still developing is socially risky (see Chapter 6 for LGBTQ+ identification). To contain the risk, adolescents use play. For example, a girl might mock-punch a boy's arm, or a boy might playfully try to put on a girls' shoe. This allows them to "save face" if the other rejects their overture. This is known as "poke-and-push courtship." As heterosexual interests develop, youth follow a typical progression: First, they attend mixed-gender activities (e.g., school dances), then group date (e.g., going to a movie together), then short-lived two-person dating, then longer-term romance. This long progression often starts around age 14–15, but ages vary widely with some starting earlier, others later.

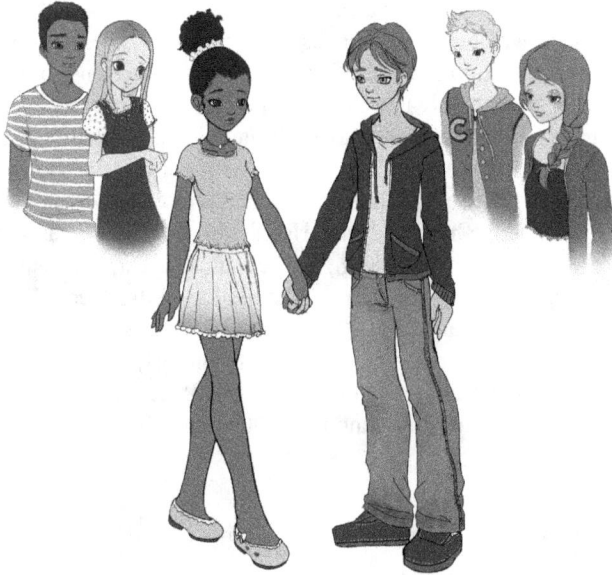

Figure 5.1 Some adolescents develop romantic relationships that can affect their social–emotional competence.

Is romance good for adolescents? Mostly not. Romance can bring stress and conflict that adolescents cannot yet manage. Teens who date regularly tend to do more poorly in school and are at higher risk for depression, victimization, and substance use. Some even report being physically assaulted (10%) or psychologically abused (25%) on a date in the past year (Foshee et al., 2009). On the other hand, romantic partners can function like an attachment relationship, providing feelings of security and comfort (Gómez-López et al., 2019). However, these benefits of romance are more likely to occur in young adulthood rather than adolescence (see Chapter 6).

Early Sexual Activity

Most (62%) high-school students have never been sexually active. A minority (38%) have had sex at least once, most (60%) of whom say they wished they had waited (Centers for Disease Control, 2020). About 15% are promiscuous, having unprotected sex with multiple partners (Inanc et al., 2020). Boys are more likely to initiate sex early and to have more partners than girls. Girls are less likely to be satisfied with their sexual debut experience and more likely to experience unwanted sex.

A key concern for early sexual activity is the risk of sexually transmitted infections (STIs), which can become diseases (STDs). Adolescent relationships tend to be short-lived, which could lead sexually active teens to have several partners, which greatly increases the risk of STIs. A quarter of sexually active adolescent girls may have STIs, making it an epidemic (Liddon et al., 2022). Adolescents who engage in early sexual activity tend to do poorly in school and use alcohol or other drugs. It is part of a pattern called *delinquency*. Teens who are sexually active have the same risk factors as for other aspects of anti-social behavior discussed above (e.g., insecure attachment, not living with both parents, not religious, poor emotion regulation, low self-esteem, deviant peers, negative role models; Inanc et al., 2020). Again, those with more risk factors and fewer protective factors are most at risk. In contrast, adolescents who delay sexual activity are more likely to graduate from high school (for girls), be more satisfied with their relationships, and have a lower rate of divorce in adulthood (Rotz et al., 2020).

Development of the Self in Adolescence

Self-Control

Self-control refers to intentional control over your actions to pursue future-oriented, long-term goals. It involves controlling your attention, initiating action (e.g., study for a test you really don't want to), and inhibiting action (e.g., don't say something mean to a friend when you are angry). Adolescents continue to increase in self-control compared to younger children. They are able to persist on complex, long-term projects, or delay gratification for a long time (e.g., saving money to buy a car). This is partly due to development of a part of the brain (the prefrontal cortex) that makes advanced thinking possible. However, in adolescence, the part of the brain that responds to reward matures faster than the part of the brain that stops impulsive behavior. This means teens still need guidance from adults. Some people also think this means that teens are more likely to take risks than at any other age. This is not the case for most youth, but those who are more reward-seeking and/or have low self-control do take more risks. However, this is not just the case for adolescents; younger children and emerging adults who are especially reward-seeking and/or have low self-control also take more risks. Youth who have low self-control are also more likely to have mental health challenges, be less prosocial, and more antisocial. They tend to have trouble controlling their temper, are easily distracted, are hyperactive, and have few plans for important goals.

What leads to high self-control in youth? Key causes are inductive discipline and authoritative parenting (see Chapter 4). Unfortunately, some parents who used power assertion when their children were younger, shift to psychological control when their children become adolescents. It is difficult to use power assertion when youth are acquiring their own resources (e.g., money) and are as big as the parents, so some parents switch to psychological control through emotional manipulation. For example, if a teen hurts a parent's feelings, the parent stops talking to their child until the child pleases them again. Parents who increase psychological control of their teens tend to have teens who decrease in *self*-control (and increase in aggression, drug use, and truancy) because psychological control is coercive and undermines teen's autonomy. Other factors that undermine self-control include media use, adversity, and toxic stress.

Self-Esteem

In Chapter 4, you learned that healthy self-esteem comes from secure attachment and feelings of competence. You also learned that middle-school children are more accurate than preschoolers at judging their own competence, which may result in *decreased* self-esteem. Adolescents continue this downward trend, possibly because their assessment of their ability becomes even more accurate. Youth are constantly compared with others, such as in competitive sports, grading in school, and social interaction. Thus, self-esteem tends to decrease from age 10 to about 15, but then starts to increase (Rimm-Kaufman et al., 2024).

Within these general age trends, some adolescents have higher self-esteem than others. Higher self-esteem is linked to greater happiness, better mental and physical health, and greater likelihood of graduating from college and having stable employment. In contrast, in adolescence low self-esteem is linked to depression, anxiety, and delinquency. Although high self-esteem is related to positive outcomes, it is not clear whether raising self-esteem then causes these positive outcomes or whether positive events in life cause high self-esteem.

Ironically, youth can have too much or unrealistically high self-esteem. Bullies often think they are entitled or justified in harming others because they are superior. Yet, their high self-esteem may be brittle. They may harm others in order to defend their brittle self-esteem. Brittle self-esteem can also be manifest in perfectionism, workaholic behavior, and showing off wealth. Narcissistic personality disorder is a mental condition in which people have an inflated sense of their own importance, a deep need for excessive attention and admiration, troubled relationships, and a lack of empathy for others. But, behind this mask of extreme confidence lies a fragile self-esteem that is vulnerable to the slightest criticism. Youth with genuinely healthy self-esteem are not threatened by attacks on their ego.

Personality and Identity

In Chapter 4, you learned there is a general age trend toward more positive personality traits across time. This is true during adolescence, when youth on average become more extraverted and emotionally stable. One exception is that in early adolescence there may be a temporary dip in agreeableness, openness, and conscientiousness. By mid-adolescence, on average, youth tend to increase in these three attributes and continue to do so into young adulthood. Within individuals, positive traits tend to be more stable than negative traits. This means that conscientious and agreeable youth tend to continue to have the same traits as adults.

Identity Exploration and Development

Personality is a pattern of broad traits (dispositions, characteristics), goals, values, motives, and self-defining life narratives, situated within one's culture and social context. Identity is part of personality and includes a view of the self: Who am I? Who will I be in the future? What does my life mean? We create stories about ourselves that integrate our past and our imagined future. These *self-narratives* that make up our identity are initially based on conversations with parents about causes and consequences of events in our lives. Until about age 10, children believe that their parents know more about them than they know about themselves. In adolescence, youth begin to take ownership of their own self-narratives. Our self-narratives are not entirely aligned with reality, but rather represent how we choose to remember and understand our lives.

Some psychologists (Marcia, 2002) propose stages of identity development in the following order:

1. Foreclosure. In this stage, teens accept their identity as it is given to them from external sources such as parents and peers without questioning, wondering, or exploring. The opening vignette shows the power of a teacher, as a person of authority, in shaping Nicole and Mitch's adolescent identities.
2. Moratorium. This is a period of discovery as teens search out their own identity in their own words, ask questions, and explore.
3. Identity achievement. Teens commit to an adaptive, coherent identity.

If an adaptive identity is not achieved, then *identity diffusion* occurs. This means adolescents try-on many roles, struggle to commit to specific roles, and lack clarity about goals and values. Identity diffusion is linked to maladaptive outcomes for youth.

Adolescents' identity can focus on their relationships (e.g., son, sister, boyfriend), economic status, gender, sexual orientation, culture/ethnicity/race, religion, competence, and other domains. The self becomes more diverse with age, which in middle adolescence can lead to conflicted identity if different roles have contradictory attributes. For example, a girl might think she is "friendly toward others," but mean girls in her school have forced her to behave like an introvert, which she says is not "the real me." However, by late adolescence, most youth are able to integrate seemingly contradictory selves. They come to understand it is reasonable and adaptive to act differently in different situations.

Gender Identity

In Chapter 3, you learned that young children tend to be highly gender stereotyping, but this diminishes through middle childhood. However, there is an uptick again in gender stereotyping in adolescence, such as "boys are better at math than girls." Youth who fit the stereotypes for their gender tend to fare well, unless they feel too much pressure to conform to stereotypes. However, emotionally healthy youth are also more likely to feel they can try out activities typical of the other gender if they want to. Feeling content with one's gender, and typical of one's gender, are linked to social–emotional well-being.

Ethnic Identity

In Chapter 4, you learned having a healthy ethnic/racial identity helps protect youth from negative experiences of discrimination, leading to better success in school and social–emotional well-being. But, you also learned that racist events can undermine children's emotional well-being. In adolescence, racism can place youth at greater risk for behavior problems, risky sex, substance use, poor sleep, delinquency, and crime. Box 5.2 illustrates a mixed-ethnicity adolescent who has navigated a positive self-identity.

Box 5.2   Identity Case Study

Everette is a high-school junior. He has been educated in private schools since preschool. His current school has a heavy emphasis on academics and some emphasis on social–emotional learning (SEL). His school environment is predominantly White, but he is of mixed ethnicity. He describes his life as stable because his family is stable. His parents are married and he is an only child. His parents are older than many of his friends' parents.

He has faced some challenges, such as being born prematurely. He has some learning differences that he copes with through his own efforts and help from others. He acknowledges some emotion regulation and communication problems when he gets angry. This happens mostly when people do not understand him.

Everette has specific goals for the near future. He sees the value of education, which his parents stress. He also wants to maintain his fitness and have a career where he can help people in some way. He wants to get

---

a bachelor's degree. Being an only child with school friends who live far away, he doesn't get as much social interaction as he would like, but he believes he is socially well adjusted and able to maintain good relationships. In the future, he hopes to meet people who are like him, and he would like to experience more varied social situations.

Overall, he believes he is socially and emotionally competent because he gets good feedback from his peers, parents, and other adults. He feels successful in his life. He feels his parents, his teachers, and his school environment made him who he is. He also believes that his spiritual beliefs have had some influence over who he is.

Strategies to Foster Social–Emotional Competence in Adolescence

To promote social–emotional competence in adolescence, you will use some of the same strategies discussed in Chapters 3 and 4, so review the sections on strategies in those chapters. That is: (1) form attachment-like relationships in which youth feel safe to learn and fail, (2) use inductive discipline to help them learn acceptable behavior, (3) be authoritative, (4) increase prosocial behavior, (5) talk about emotions, (6) create a primarily emotionally positive environment, but express an array of emotions, (7) coach coping strategies, (8) convey respect and admiration to youth and help them develop valued skills so their self-esteem is healthy, (9) improve peer status, and (10) help youth develop a healthy ethnic identity. An additional way to increase prosocial behavior in youth is to help them find ways to serve their community, which is linked to greater self-esteem, acceptance of others, and bonding to the community. Finally, you can promote self-control in youth by supporting: (1) participation in religion, which presumably is linked to self-control through religions' emphasis on self-mastery and (2) parental monitoring. Children whose parents monitor them, but not in an overly controlling way, tend to have more self-control. Building social–emotional competency tends to result in other competencies because they are interrelated. For example, research has found that youth are more prosocial when they read others' emotions well because they have good theory of mind skills and they can control their own emotions rather than become easily upset or depressed. Youth who are well-liked are prosocial, empathic, and good at perspective-taking.

How Does Sleep Contribute to Social–Emotional Competence?

Adults in any role who work with adolescents should be aware of sleep deprivation, which is an epidemic among today's youth. Sleep deprivation symptoms masquerade as social–emotional problems, including ADHD, anxiety, and depression. Sleep deprivation and emotional disorders are bidirectional, meaning each can cause the other. Youth with unhealthy sleep habits – such as sleeping less than 7 hours a night or having more than a 2-hour difference between school-night and weekend bedtimes – tend to be more depressed than other children. You do not have to feel sleepy for sleep deprivation to have these effects. Adolescents who experience mental health issues often need more sleep than the recommended amount. You can promote adolescents' social–emotional well-being by teaching them good sleep habits and creating conditions that promote adequate amounts of sleep (e.g., do not hold events late at night).

How Can You Help Youth Improve Perspective-Taking?

Adolescents tend to falsely believe that how they perceive the world is correct, rather than a perception that is filtered by their motives, experiences, and expectations. This unconscious bias is part of being a human, but it can lead to self-deception or self-protection that is not good for them or those around them. When teens are taught that everyone has this bias to some extent and are given the opportunity to listen to peers who have different perspectives, they can improve their ability to take the perspective of others, increase empathizing with others, and reduce social anxiety about being negatively evaluated by their peers (Smith, 2020). For example, if a clerk at a store is curt with them, instead of responding with anger, they might think the clerk is having a bad day or that they "took that the wrong way." This is the reappraisal coping strategy.

How Can You Help Youth Who Are Depressed?

Above, you learned that depression is common in youth, with prevalence peaking around 15–17 years, and that mental health issues begin, or worsen, during adolescence. Youth with depression should receive professional help (see Chapters 8–11). While they are receiving this help, other adults in their world can help by doing the same things you would do to help any youth develop healthy emotion regulation skills. This includes teaching good coping strategies, creating an emotionally positive environment, talking about emotions (especially gratitude), using inductive discipline, and creating secure attachment-like relationships.

Chapter Summary

During adolescence, youth improve in emotion regulation. Teens are more likely than younger children to use constructive coping strategies, particularly *reappraisal,* to regulate their emotions. Emotionally healthy teens tend to have more positive than negative emotions, but not *only* positive emotions.

Adolescents continue to improve in reading others' emotions, though they do not generally increase in empathy. Attachment continues to be important for adolescents, although attachment behaviors change. Even though secure adolescents may sometimes avoid their parents, they become independent because of secure attachment.

Adolescents are more skilled at prosocial behavior compared to younger children, but they are *not more frequently* prosocial. Aggression steadily declines from preschool to adulthood with the exception of a temporary spike in middle school. *Adolescent-onset* antisocial behavior tends to die out with age, but *childhood-onset* antisocial behavior tends to predict long-term problems. Perceived popular youth may have high social status for a time, but they tend to become troubled as they age.

Adolescence is a time of identity exploration that follows a series of stages. Gender segregation during middle childhood evolves into more mixed-gender groups in high school. Romance may develop, though teens who date regularly tend to have more negative outcomes. Early sexual activity predicts poor outcomes and can lead to STDs. Teens tend to be sleep deprived, and sleep deprivation is related to poor social–emotional development as well as academic problems.

Suggested Readings

Damour, L. (2023). *The emotional lives of teenagers: Raising connected, capable, and compassionate adolescents*. Ballantine.

Morris, A., Criss, M., Silk, J., & Houltberg, B. (2017). The impact of parenting on emotion regulation during childhood and adolescence. *Child Development Perspectives*, *11*(4), 233–238.

References

Bergin, C. (2018). *Designing a prosocial classroom: Fostering collaboration in students from pre-K-12 with the curriculum you already use*. Norton.

Bianchi, D., Lonigro, A., Baiocco, R., Baumgartner, E., & Laghi, F. (2020). Social anxiety and peer communication quality during adolescence: The interaction of social avoidance, empathic concern and perspective taking. *Child and Youth Care Forum, 49*, 853–876. https://doi.org/10.1007/s10566-020-09562-S

Bussey, K., Quinn, C., & Dobson, J. (2015). The moderating role of empathic concern and perspective taking on the relationship between moral disengagement and aggression. *Merrill-Palmer Quarterly, 61*(1), 10–29.

Centers for Disease Control (CDC). (2020). Trends in the Prevalence of Sexual Behaviors and HIV Testing National YRBS: 1991—2019 (CDC, Division of Adolescent and School Health, National Center for HIV/AIDS, Viral Hepatitis, STD, and TB Prevention, Issue. www.cdc.gov/healthyyouth/data/yrbs/factsheets/2019_sexual_trend_yrbs.htm

Cole, V. T., Richmond-Rakerd, L. S., Bierce, L. F., Norotsky, R. L., Peiris, S. T., & Hussong, A. M. (2024). Peer connectedness and substance use in adolescence: A systematic review and meta-analysis. *Psychology of Addictive Behaviors*, *38*(1), 19.

Coyne, S. M., Warburton, W., Essig, L. W., & Stockdale, L. (2018). Violent video games, externalizing behavior, and prosocial behavior: A five-year longitudinal study during adolescence. *Developmental Psychology*, *54*(10), 1868–1880. https://doi.org/10.1037/dev0000574

Curlee, A. S., Aiken, L. S., & Luthar, S. S. (2019). Middle school peer reputation in high-achieving schools: Ramifications for maladjustment versus competence by age 18. *Development and Psychopathology*, *31*, 683–697. https://doi.org/10.1017/S09545 79418000275

Foshee, V. A., Benefield, T., Suchindran, C., Ennett, S., Bauman, K. E., Karriker-Jaffe, K. J., Reyes, H., & Mathias, J. (2009). The development of four types of adolescent dating abuse and selected demographic correlates. *Journal of Research on Adolescence*, *19*(3), 380–400.

Gómez-López, M., Viejo, C., & Ortega-Ruiz, R. (2019). Well-being and romantic relationships: A systematic review in adolescence and emerging adulthood. *International Journal of Environmental Research and Public Health*, *16*(13), 2415–2446. https://doi.org/10.3390/ijerph16132415

Gutman, L. M., Peck, S. C., Malanchuk, O., Sameroff, A. J., & Eccles, J. S. (2017). VII: Problem behaviors. *Monographs of the Society for Research in Child Development*, *82*(4), 106–113. https://doi.org/10.1111/mono.12333

Inanc, H., Meckstroth, A., Keating, B., Adamek, K., Zaveri, H., O'Neil, S., McDonald, K., & Ochoa, L. (2020). *Factors influencing youth sexual activity: Conceptual models for sexual risk avoidance and cessation.* OPRE Research Brief #2020-153. U.S. Department of Health and Human Services.

Jankowski, K., & Pfeifer, J. (2021). Self-conscious emotion processing in autistic adolescents: Over-reliance on learned social rules during tasks with heightened perspective-taking demands may serve as compensatory strategy for less reflexive mentalizing. *Journal of Autism and Developmental Disorders*, *51*, 3514–3532. https://doi.org/10.1007/s10803-020-04808-6

Lam, C. B., McHale, S. M., & Crouter, A. C. (2014). Time with peers from middle childhood to late adolescence: Developmental course and adjustment correlates. *Child Development*, *85*(4), 1677–1693. https://doi.org/10.1111/cdev.12235

Liddon, N., Pampati, S., Dunville, R., Kilmer, G., & Steiner, R. J. (2022). Annual STI testing among sexually active adolescents. *Pediatrics*, *149*(5). https://doi.org/10.1542/peds.2021-051893

Marcia, J. E. (2002). Identity and psychosocial development in adulthood. *Identity: An International Journal of Theory and Research*, *2*(1), 7–28.

Musu, L., Zhang, A., Wang, K., Zhang, J., & Oudekerk, B. A. (2019). *Indicators of School Crime and Safety: 2018.*

Rimm-Kaufman, S. E., Soland, J., & Kuhfeld, M. (2024). Social and emotional competency development from fourth to 12th grade: Relations to parental education and gender. *American Psychologist* (advanced online publication). https://doi.org/10.1037/amp0001357

Rotz, D., Goesling, B., Redel, N., Shiferaw, M., & Smither-Wulsin, C. (2020). *Assessing the Benefits of Delayed Sexual Activity: A Synthesis of the Literature* (OPRE Report # 2020-04).

Silvers, J. A. (2022). Adolescence as a pivotal period for emotion regulation development. *Current Opinion in Psychology, 44,* 258–263. https://doi.org/10.1016/j.copsyc.2021.09.023

Smith, S. (2020). Teaching further education students the effects of naive realism, to support social development and mitigate classroom conflict. *Educational & Child Psychology, 37*(3), 36–68.

Chapter 6

Social and Emotional Competence in Emerging Adulthood (Ages 19–25)

Eduardo is working as a swim coach for the community youth team while attending college. He works hard to become a better coach. He is currently working on what he calls "sandwich" feedback, meaning to tell swimmers what they did well, then what they need to improve, followed by more positive reinforcement. "I liked how you did your turns. Let's work on proper head movements now. I noticed that you increased your speed." He makes a point of celebrating each improvement of individual swimmers. The kids feel like he really cares about them. Eduardo loves his work but hopes to become a coach for Olympic hopefuls after he finishes college. He is grateful that he can live at home while he is paying for college.

Eduardo has positive goals as he is entering the workforce and a strong identity. The way his team feels about him suggests he has good social–emotional competencies. What factors have supported his well-being as he has left adolescence and is now an adult? In this chapter, you will learn about emerging adulthood.

Emerging adulthood refers to the period from about age 19 to 25 (although some consider it 18–29). The body continues to mature, with changes in muscle and fat mass; young men will complete puberty during this period (girls typically complete it in adolescence). Legal status changes in ways that can alter the trajectory of one's life course – individuals can serve in the military, be tried as adults, consume alcohol, and get married without parental consent.

A key aspect of this age is *self-sufficiency*. Indeed, some define "adulthood" as accepting responsibility for one's self, making independent decisions, and assuming financial independence (Arnett, 2015). Emerging adults leave compulsory schooling, and many transition to living independently from parents while starting career paths. In the USA, roughly 40% pursue work and 60% enter college (many do a combination of both, like Eduardo). It is common to change college majors or career paths during this time. In addition, most will also enter long-term relationships including marriage and parenthood, although recent generations are delaying marriage. In the USA, the median age at first marriage is now 28 (women) and 30 (men), compared to 22 and 24 in 1980.

DOI: 10.4324/9781003046455-6

Emerging adulthood is an exciting period of life full of possibilities, but because big decisions are made at this age – such as careers and marriage – it can also be intimidating. Facing such big decisions activates another key aspect of this age, which is *identity exploration*. This is related to the stages of identity development discussed in Chapter 5. Some emerging adults feel they are in-between childhood and independence, but still lacking many adult skills, and experiencing a lot of instability with frequent changes in living arrangement, relationships, work, and schooling.

Development of Emotional Competence in Emerging Adulthood

The transition to higher education or the workforce presents both challenges and opportunities for emotional development. Positive experiences that foster autonomy and provide support can enhance individuals' emotion regulation skills.

Emotion Regulation

In Chapter 5, you learned that by age 10, emotionally healthy children will have near adult-like ability to regulate their own emotions, although ability to use coping strategies, especially reappraisal, grows in adolescence. Thus, there are not dramatic changes in emotion regulation in emerging adulthood on average. However, there are large individual differences in emotion regulation. Individuals with good emotion regulation tend to have greater workplace success, like Eduardo. The term "emotional intelligence" was coined in a popular book that claimed it is more important for workplace success than IQ. Follow-on research found that this claim was overstated; nevertheless, emotional competence does contribute to success after accounting for IQ and personality.

In contrast, individuals who experience adversity, insecure attachment, or social–emotional challenges carried over from childhood now face big life decisions for which they do not have adequate support and are not prepared, making it hard to move toward self-sufficiency. Thus, it is not surprising that substance use and feelings of isolation peak at this age, about two to four times higher in emerging adulthood than adolescence. Roughly, 75% of lifetime cases of mental disorders will begin by age 24 (Kessler et al., 2005). First episodes of psychosis (hallucinations, delusions) typically occur in the early 20s. Roughly, 14% of emerging adults will experience serious mental disorders (e.g., bipolar, schizophrenia, major depression). However, keep in mind that this means most emerging adults do not have serious mental disorders.

Some individual emerging adults have better emotion regulation than others. What might influence these differences? Just as at younger ages, parenting quality plays a crucial role. Parents need to continue as attachment figures (AFs), and they need to support the child leading an *independent* life. When mothers experience secure attachment with their emerging adult children, the children tend to have good mental health and exhibit prosocial behavior. Parents who are warm and model use of reappraisal as a coping strategy have emerging adult children who are better at reappraisal, a mature coping strategy. In contrast, parents who use psychological control (see Chapter 4) hinder their emerging adult children's emotion regulation. Sometimes, parents need a professional's help navigating their role with an emerging adult child because the relationship shifts when their children leave the nest. When parents have their own mental health challenges, it is difficult for emerging adult children to become independent. Thus, an emerging adult may need a professional's help to recognize whether the parent–child relationship is healthy and how to navigate it so they can become successful adults. As interview Box 6.1 illustrates, taking courses in human development may also help.

Reading Other's Emotions (Affective Perspective-Taking)

In contrast to emotion regulation, which does not change much, the ability to read others' emotions continues to grow substantially across adulthood. Emerging adults are better at reading others' emotions compared to adolescents, probably due to more experience with other people. They are better able to consider motives in other people. For example, if Mary does not like Eugenia, why does she invite Eugenia to a party? Why does she tell everyone that Eugenia is great? What ulterior motives might she have?

Box 6.1   Interview with a Professor

Karina is an emeritus professor with 32 years of experience in child development. She enhances the social–emotional competence of emerging adults by teaching them how to have good family relationships, good friendships, and good intimate relationships. Karina believes that social–emotional competence is one of the most precious characteristics and skills for all humans at all developmental points.

Development of Social Competence in Emerging Adulthood

A key component of social competence is feeling connected to others. In 2023, the Surgeon General of the USA issued an advisory about the epidemic of loneliness and lack of connection to others. It states, "This decline [in time spent with friends] is starkest for young people ages 15 to 24. For this age group, time spent in-person with friends has reduced by nearly 70% over almost two decades, from roughly 150 minutes per day in 2003 to 40 minutes per day in 2020" (U.S. Surgeon General, 2023, p. 13). While the COVID-19 pandemic accelerated trends in shrinking social interaction, the trend existed *prior* to COVID-19. In addition, family size and marriage rates have declined, the number of people who live alone has doubled since 1960, and people belong to fewer organizations, including religious institutions. This means people have fewer informal and formal communities of social support. This is a problem because social connection predicts several important outcomes: physical health, education, mental health, prosperity, and overall well-being. In this section, we discuss key elements of social competence and connectedness.

Attachment

Secure attachment continues to be important in emerging adulthood because parents' support of their children's independence helps children become self-sufficient. Recall that secure AFs provide a base from which children, including emerging adults, explore the world. During emerging adulthood, as in adolescence, parents are typically primary AFs, but peers can serve as secondary AFs. When emerging adults experience a crisis, they often turn first to their AFs for help or advice. Emerging adults can be independent if they feel secure and know they can call on parents for support and guidance when needed.

In emerging adults, secure attachment to parents is linked to increased self-esteem, emotion regulation, coping skills, empathy, and prosocial behavior – and decreased depression, anxiety, stress, and aggression. Secure attachment to a primary AF predicts secure attachment to peers, which predicts better mental health. This pattern holds because models of healthy relationships learned from parents get applied to peers. This goes for romantic relationships as well. Parent–child attachment relationships become self-fulfilling prophecies that continue to influence social relationships over time.

In adulthood, whether one's attachment is secure or not is measured using the *Adult Attachment Interview* (AAI). This interview involves asking you to list five adjectives that describe your relationship with each parent, and to describe specific incidents that illustrate that adjective. *Secure* individuals are able to: (1) discuss the relationship in a coherent way, (2) describe parents' positive and negative influence, and (3) value the relationship. *Insecure* individuals may either dismiss the importance of relationships ("My dad and I didn't get along, but it doesn't matter") or idealize their parents ("They are the best!") while describing negative memories that contradict the claim that their parents are the best. For example, they may describe events of significant rejection (e.g., being kicked out of the house) as not being a big deal. Or, they may ramble, provide excessively detailed descriptions. Or, they may suddenly become silent during the AAI, as though they are at a loss for describing the relationship. They may communicate strong anger or fear when talking about a parent, or a preoccupation with trying to please the parent.

Attachment is typically stable from infancy to adulthood, but it can change if family functioning and parents' sensitivity improves or deteriorates. This can happen as a result of events in childhood, such as parents' divorce. Parental divorce in childhood can negatively influence emerging adults' ability to form their own stable romantic relationships. Attachment can also change as a result of big events during young adulthood, such as losing a job or getting married. When life stabilizes, young adults are likely to revert to their security of attachment prior to the big event, but they could also have long-term change.

Prosocial Behavior

Emerging adults have expanded opportunity to be prosocial as they become acquainted with more and different kinds of people. Emerging adults who are more prosocial have many benefits including:

1. *More positive relationships and better social networks*. People prefer to be with someone who is kind, humble, and helpful. In Chapter 3, you learned that preference for prosocial others begins in infancy and continues into adulthood. Prosocial behavior is among the most important factors in adult's impressions of one another, and it is *the most sought-after attribute in a romantic partner* (Goodwin, 2015; Thomas et al., 2020). There may be a small gender difference in this preference, in that adult women value care and fairness somewhat more than men and may be more concerned when care or fairness is violated.
2. *Greater mental health* (especially less depression), happiness, sense of well-being, life satisfaction, self-acceptance, and personal growth (Nelson et al., 2016). This occurs across cultures. An added bonus is that the recipients of prosocial behavior get a bigger boost in happiness than you might expect.
3. *Preparation for college and career success*. Like Eduardo, prosocial emerging adults tend to have greater success in their jobs than those who lack prosocial skills whether they go to college or not. In college, prosocial students are better participants in groupwork, which prepares them for workplace collaboration. Time spent by workers in collaborative activities has increased by 50% or more over the last 2 decades because people who work in teams tend to achieve better results and report higher job satisfaction (Atwell, 2023). In the workplace, prosocial employees are in high demand by employers. The World Economic Forum has stated that jobs in today's global economy increasingly require prosocial skills such as the ability to collaborate. Among the skills that best predict workforce success are social skills, self-control, and healthy self-esteem. A vice president of American Airlines said that

her quarter-century as a business executive taught her that people who are kind and empathetic are better to work with than people with a high IQ and impressive credentials.

The same factors that influence whether individuals are prosocial in childhood pertain to emerging adults, with the biggest being family influences, particularly attachment to mothers. Emerging adults' degree of prosocial behavior is also influenced by their media use, by their peer relationships if they provide opportunities for practicing prosocial behavior and receiving social reinforcement, and by their culture. Prosocial behavior is valued widely across cultures, but some cultures may promote norms of group harmony more than others and provide more opportunity to practice prosocial habits.

Antisocial Behavior

In Chapter 5, you learned that youth who are temporarily delinquent during adolescence tend to outgrow it by adulthood, but those with childhood-onset aggression tend to have long-term problems. Although some of them will decrease aggression in adulthood, those who continue to be aggressive can get into serious trouble because behaviors that were tolerated in children, like hurting someone, are considered criminal by age 18. Indeed, individuals with *childhood*-onset antisocial behavior are more likely than those with *adolescent*-onset to engage in criminal activity at age 20. They also tend to have other adult problems, such as lower-status jobs, unemployment, drug use, drunk driving, marriage/partner problems, divorce, premature parenthood, and harsh parenting of their own children, thus creating intergenerational cycles of antisocial behavior. Fortunately, emerging adults can break these intergenerational cycles with intervention from the kind of professionals that we'll discuss in Chapters 8–11.

Just as with prosocial behavior, a primary predictor of antisocial behavior is parenting. Parents who have low levels of self-control and high levels of conflict are more likely to have emerging adult children who are antisocial. If parents learn to provide consistent discipline, use induction, and provide emotional support, their children are less likely to become antisocial. Negative peer influences, such as association with delinquent friends, can exacerbate antisocial behavior in emerging adults. Furthermore, stress related to low income, such as violence in the neighborhood and limited access to resources, predicts increased antisocial behavior. Finally, cultural norms regarding aggression and social behavior influence antisocial behavior, such as community beliefs about what constitutes antisocial behavior or the criminal justice system's approach to juvenile delinquency that can either remediate or solidify antisocial behavior.

Today, one source of aggression, even for those who are not in intergenerational cycles of aggression, is violent media. Emerging adults who are exposed to violent models in movies, videogames, comic books, and song lyrics are more aggressive. For example, in one study, college students were randomly assigned to play a violent or a nonviolent videogame for 25 minutes per day. They were then shown violent photos (e.g., a man holding a gun to another person's head). Scans of their brains showed less response to the violent photos if they had played violent games. They were also given an opportunity to play a competitive game afterwards. Those who played violent games were more aggressive during the game. This study looked at what happens right after playing a violent video game. But, the participants who reported often playing video games *before* the experiment also had less brain response to violent photos (Engelhardt et al., 2011).)

Theory of Mind

Theory of mind continues to develop through young adulthood. Emerging adults are better than adolescents at understanding sarcasm, making persuasive arguments, negotiating, and enjoying witty humor. However, just like adolescents, emerging adults sometimes make mistakes, assume people know the same things they know, or have the same interests they have. At age 80, you will have better theory of mind than you have at age 20.

Conflict Resolution

There are three ways that conflict can be resolved: coercion, disengagement (e.g., leave the conflict situation), and compromise. Not until emerging adulthood are conflicts more often resolved with compromise. At younger ages, children say they prefer compromise in hypothetical situations, but in actual conflict, they may resort to coercion. One exception is taking turns, which younger children are able to do on their own. Thus, preference for compromise does not actually become behavior until emerging adulthood.

Romance

Romance is a key developmental task of emerging adulthood. In Chapter 5, you learned that early romance can start during adolescence. However, many individuals do not become involved in romance until later, with 20% having no romantic relationship before age 25. Specific dating patterns have been called continuous singles, late starters, moderate daters, and frequent changers (Gonzalez Avilés et al., 2021). You may know people who fit each pattern.

In Chapter 5, you also learned that in adolescence, early romance can be beneficial but is more likely to be a source of stress, depression, and anxiety. In contrast, romance is more likely to be beneficial in young adulthood because relationships tend to be more supportive and longer term. Romantic partners can function like an attachment relationship, providing feelings of security and comfort. Individuals have better mental health and greater well-being in committed relationships with mutual relationship satisfaction. High-quality relationships are characterized by commitment, shared goals, interdependency, clear communication, shared positive experiences and emotions, power equality, partner idealization, intimacy, and prosocial behavior (e.g., apologizing, forgiveness, helping, gratitude). Individuals in marriage (after age 22) tend to fare better than those in co-habitation or other relationship types (Gómez-López et al., 2019). Thus, romance, particularly marriage, can be a protective factor in young adulthood, if it is a high-quality relationship.

Most emerging adults will have more than one dating (but not necessarily sexual) partner before they marry, if they marry. This means that "breaking up" is common. Break-ups are linked to depression, anxiety, stress, and victimization (Gómez-López et al., 2019). The brain processes this "hurt" in the same way it processes physical pain. In one study, the brains were scanned of adults who had recently broken-up with a romantic partner while they looked at pictures of their "ex" and thought about their break-up. Then, they were given a physical pain test (intense heat on their arm). In both situations, the same area in their brains became active (Kross et al., 2011). Furthermore, pain relievers, like Tylenol, reduce the pain of social rejection.

Whether you have high-quality, stable romantic relationships is linked to social–emotional competence – particularly less aggression and more prosocial behavior, empathy, emotion regulation, constructive coping strategies, theory of mind skills, and self-control (Gómez-López et al., 2019). You won't be surprised that a stable romantic relationship is also predicted by how you were parented in childhood. As early as 3 years of age, whether you had secure attachment to your parents statistically predicts the security of your romantic relationships, even 60 years later (Waldinger & Schulz, 2016).

Securely attached emerging adults tend to have stable, long-term romantic relationships that are trusting, committed, and independent. They serve as a secure base to their partners: openly expressing worries, receiving reassurance, seldom arguing, feeling intimacy, and not threatening to leave. Compared to insecure couples, secure couples have fewer arguments, greater intimacy, and fewer breakups.

Research finds different types of insecure adult attachment in romantic relationships. *Insecure anxious* adults tend to be jealous, worry that their partner will leave, and lack trust in their partners, yet they anxiously seek to be in relationships. They are eager to share personal information and to fall in love. They frequently break-up and reunite. Their strong need to avoid abandonment can lead them to be clingy and suffocating to their partners. They may try to make their partner jealous, which can create *more* anxiety. *Insecure avoidant* adults tend to be uncomfortable with closeness and fear being smothered. They want freedom and control over their time. This pattern of behavior often pushes partners away. They may feel that they don't need others.

Not only does your early attachment history influence later romantic relationships but so does the way you were *disciplined*. For example, in one study 13-year-olds whose parents used psychological control to discipline them had less supportive romantic relationships at age 27 and lower likelihood of being in a relationship by age 32 (Loeb et al., 2021).

The quality of romantic relationships can be changed; if you had an insecure attachment to parents, you are not doomed to difficult relationships. Everyone is capable of developing relationship skills, for example through clinical therapy (see Chapters 10 and 11). Furthermore, marriages are the formation of new attachment relationships. If someone with an insecure attachment history to their parents marries someone with a secure attachment history, they may become secure in the marriage. (Note that this may not be as common in non-married romantic partnerships which tend to be shorter-lived compared to marriages.) Individuals who are securely attached to *both* their parents and to their spouse tend to have the most stable and satisfying relationships. Do you recognize different patterns of adult attachment in your friends' romantic relationships?

Sexual and Gender Minority (LGBTQ+)

Most adults (80%–95%) are heterosexual, but the age group most likely to identify as non-heterosexual (up to 15% in the USA) is emerging adulthood. Non-heterosexual young adults may identify as lesbian, gay, bisexual, transgender, questioning, or in other ways (LGBTQ+). This means that they are attracted to either their own sex or to both sexes, or they do not identify with the gender they were assigned at birth (Bailey et al., 2016). Gender minority females are more likely than males to change in sexual attraction over time. Trans-youth may identify as the opposite sex as early as middle childhood, and some begin to identify in adolescence, although more research is needed (Hässler et al., 2022).

Most LGBTQ+ individuals experience social–emotional well-being. However, some may be victims of bullying or peer rejection, which can make it difficult to establish high-quality friendships. This can lead to spending more time alone and less involvement in social activities, which can lead to higher risk of depression, suicide, substance use, risky sex, violence, and strained family relationships.

Research on the causes of LGBTQ+ orientation has suggested several possible factors including perinatal experiences (i.e., hormone exposure during pregnancy, low birthweight, shortened breastfeeding time, following the birth of older brothers) and parenting factors (i.e., abuse, absent parents, or poor parent–child relationships) (Ablaza et al., 2022; Bailey et al., 2016; Xu et al., 2019).

There may be inherited tendency toward gay male sexual orientation, but the evidence is not clear and is even less so for female orientation.

Cultural Competence

Cultural competence, also called *multicultural competence*, involves being open-minded, having empathy toward and knowledge of others' cultures, and motivation and skill to connect with those in other cultures. It moves beyond mere tolerance of others who are different. Culture can refer to large groups such as whole countries or to smaller subgroups based on ethnic/racial group, national background, class, region, and religion. It can apply to small groups, such as workplaces, schools, or neighborhoods. Cultural boundaries are fuzzy rather than clear-cut. Each of us participates in multiple cultures, and we adopt aspects of new cultures that we are exposed to.

Cultural humility is challenging for most of us. It is natural to be biased to favor one's own culture or those similar to our own. It is easy to believe that our own culture is best, and other cultures are strange, inferior, or wrong. People may go through stages from denying differences (one's own culture is the only "real" one), to being defensive (devaluing other cultures), to minimization of differences (only seeing superficial differences), to acceptance of differences, to adaptation to differences, and finally to integrating differences (Haas, 2019). We develop mature cultural humility when we are open to learning about diverse groups and are willing to self-reflect about our own values and assumptions.

Cultural competence is an asset and can cause you to feel greater psychological well-being, less stress, greater trust, and better job satisfaction. You can be a more effective teacher, social worker, nurse, and so on if you are able to listen with humility to students, clients, and patients who are different from you. If you have better perspective-taking skills, your work group is likely to have better problem-solving, cooperation, communication, trust, and satisfaction. Being part of a work team with different cultural backgrounds can lead to greater creativity and innovation when solving a problem. For this reason, employers in many countries emphasize teamwork across diverse groups.

Box 6.2   Emerging Adult Case Study

Charles is 38 years old. Here, we share his reflections on his emerging adult years after he graduated from high school. Charles has dyslexia, so school and learning are not easy for him. He wanted to be a paramedic but couldn't pass anatomy and other classes. He decided to go into construction full time and pursue education part time. He worked with concrete for several bosses for over 3 years. He finished school and got a contractor's license around the age of 26. He is a member of the Church of Jesus Christ of Latter-day Saints (Mormon) and served a mission for 2 years in Brazil. At the age of 28, he returned home. He worked for another company while he studied for his real estate license. He also met someone special and got married. By age 30, he had started his own business with a contractor and a real-estate license. His wife is an Registered Nurse. It took her approximately 6 years to complete her degree as they started a family and business together. Charles credits three things for helping him to make it through the emerging adult period of his life. (1) His religious faith. He had partially left the church but returned to it before going on a mission to Brazil and before meeting his wife. (2) His family of origin (parents and siblings) for supporting him through this time. (3) His yearning to have kids and a stable family life. Although this period was challenging for Charles, he accomplished his dreams. He now has a wife and three children and owns a successful concrete business.

Development of the Self in Emerging Adulthood

Self-Control

Box 6.2 illustrates how changes in career plans, marriage, family support and religion converged to help Charles develop self-sufficiency in emerging adulthood. Compared to adolescents, emerging adults can be even more focused on highly delayed goals (e.g., building a concrete business or starting a family, like Charles, or coaching Olympians, like Eduardo). Emerging adults with high self-control engage in less risk-taking (e.g., alcohol use, being in a car with a drunk driver, vandalism). Individuals who had high self-control as children are more likely to become adults who complete college, are employed, have better finances and health, and do not use drugs or experience family violence.

Personality and Identity

Overall, from toddlerhood to old age, there is change toward more positive personality, with the exception we discussed in Chapter 5 about a temporary dip in early adolescence. This movement toward more positive personality is termed the *maturity principle* of personality development. There is a particularly steep increase in positive personality traits in young adulthood, perhaps linked to maturing that comes from entering the workforce and romantic relationships. This personality improvement levels off after emerging adulthood, with one exception. *Emotional stability*, which is the opposite of neuroticism, continues to rise well into old age. So, you can look forward to becoming more emotionally stable as you grow older!

Identity formation is a major developmental task in emerging adulthood. Emerging adults must transition from "one who is taken care of" to "one who takes care of others." While identity formation begins in adolescence, it stabilizes in emerging adulthood. Identity becomes more complex as your social world broadens to include people who may affect your self-narratives (e.g., romantic partner or coworkers) and as you experience new types of events (e.g., moving out of the childhood home). This can cause another wave of the moratorium stage that you learned about in Chapter 5, followed by a somewhat different identity achievement. Emerging adults with the personality trait conscientiousness (see Chapter 4) are more likely than others to experience deep exploration and commitments, which leads to identity achievement (Turner et al., 2024). Young adults with more resources (e.g., income or social networks) are able to explore identity dimensions more broadly and deeply.

Self-Narratives

Culture shapes your story through patterns or rules about how you can tell and remember a story. In Chapter 5, you learned that we grow up inside our families' stories. These can be stories of redemption (e.g., overcoming adversity, finding positive meaning in negative events, nurturing others, and social mobility). For example, a family story might tell how grandma overcame religious and gender discrimination in order to go to college. This can lead us to create our own redemptive self-narratives. For example, "My school experience was very difficult, but it helped me grow stronger and face later challenges well." On the other hand, families may pass on narratives of failure and hopelessness.

Identity can continue to change in adulthood as self-narratives evolve (Turner et al., 2024). Disequilibrium, or an identity crisis, can result from big events, such as marriage, having children, death of loved ones, or disabling injury. Remediation and change are possible at any point, but they become harder the more entrenched behavior and beliefs are, especially for those who lack a coherent sense of self. It is the role of psychotherapists (see Chapters 10 and 11) to help clients reshape a self-narrative and find growth-affirming ways to narrate and understand emotionally negative events.

Emerging adults in low-income or marginalized communities may achieve a committed identity through *counternarratives* or *counterstories* that contradict the stories told about marginalized communities by the dominant culture. Counternarratives are narratives that challenge common stereotyped beliefs and promote agency to challenge oppression. For example, a young adult could be told family stories of academic success that contradict traditional stories that young Black and Latina youth drop out of high school and do not attend college. Counternarratives can foster identity achievement.

Workplace Identity

Emerging adults develop an identity of themselves in the workforce – what they want to do, which skills they have, and in what jobs they feel they belong. Workplace competence is a huge part of identity. Emerging adults with better social–emotional skills are more equiped to build strong relationships with mentors, supervisors, and peers in the workplace, as well as stronger feelings of belonging in the workplace and expanding social capital. Social capital refers to the network of relationships that provide support and/or opportunities to you. It can come from families, neighbors, classmates, teachers, mentors, and others. Emerging adults with strong workplace identity are more likely to experience success in postsecondary education, expanded access to jobs, and improved opportunities for economic mobility. See Figure 6.1.

Emerging adults may have employment attitudes that are different from their employers because of generational effects. For example, Gen Z (born between 1997 and 2012, also called iGen) are the first generation to grow up with widespread internet access and where remote employment is common. They demand more from employers, such as work–life balance and paid time-off as a "right", compared to the preceding generations. In contrast, their employers may interpret this as "lazy," "disloyal" to the workplace, and overly "entitled."

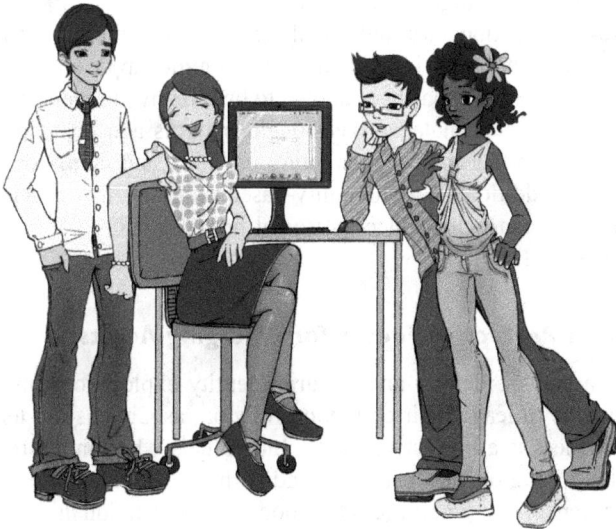

Figure 6.1 Entering the workplace or starting a career is a key developmental milestone for emerging adults.

Strategies to Foster Social–Emotional Competence in Emerging Adulthood

Review Chapter 5 for ways to foster social–emotional competence in adolescence. These same strategies apply to emerging adults. Two key factors that you have read about again and again throughout this book are secure attachment and authoritative parenting. Authoritative parents display warmth to their children and use respectful inductive discipline. Secure attachment and authoritative parenting continue to be important in emerging adulthood in order for youth to become self-sufficient adults. Authoritative parents support their emerging adult child's development of self-sufficiency because they have been scaffolding self-control since childhood.

For emerging adults who are struggling with social–emotional competence, it is more important to enhance their assets and protective factors than to try to reduce their risk factors. Enhancing assets and protective factors might involve building their prosocial behavior, mentoring them, helping them move toward personally meaningful goals, or fostering a vision of a positive future self. Some U.S. states are beginning to develop programs to meet the special needs of struggling emerging adults. For example, the state of Missouri has a website called "Life Launch" that helps improve treatment and support services for youth transitioning to adulthood who struggle with mental health. It provides advice and support as individuals move toward self-sufficiency. Online emotion regulation training programs have shown promise in improving emotion regulation abilities and overall psychological well-being.

Effective interventions for antisocial behavior in emerging adults often involve a combination of individual and systemic approaches. Cognitive-behavioral therapy (CBT) has been shown to be effective in reducing antisocial behavior by addressing maladaptive thought patterns and behaviors. Family-based interventions that improve parenting practices and family dynamics are also beneficial. Additionally, community-based programs that provide positive peer interactions can help reduce antisocial behavior. These are discussed in Chapters 10 and 11.

Is Religion a Protective Factor for Emerging Adults?

Religion is a part of identity and culture. Identity exploration can lead some emerging adults to leave their childhood religion, as Charles did temporarily. Yet, religiousness is a protective factor. Individuals who remain religious, or return to their religion like Charles, tend to have better emotion regulation from adolescence into emerging adulthood. When individuals become more religious, they tend to become more self-regulated. Perhaps this is because they are more likely to pray and meditate, which can improve self-regulation. A relationship with a divine entity can provide comfort, meaning, and peace, and reduce stress, anxiety, and depression. Religious emerging adults are more likely than non-religious to have empathy and prosocial goals of caring for others rather than personal gratification. They monitor their progress toward those goals because they feel accountable to both a higher power and to their faith community. Most religions place strong value on prosocial behaviors, such as treating others fairly, kindly, and honestly. They also provide opportunity to serve those in need, which can increase empathy. Serving others is a tenet of cultural humility training. Religious emerging adults are also less likely to prefer violent media. Violent media content, in turn, is associated with less prosocial behavior, due to reduced perspective taking and empathy. In contrast, emerging adults who prefer prosocial media (movies, internet websites) are more prosocial.

How Can You Help Emerging Adults Build Prosocial Behavior?

In addition to religious institutions, workplaces can contribute to prosocial behavior. Education and work environments that promote collaborative learning and community engagement contribute to prosocial development. Many workplaces have "wellness" programs designed to promote well-being in employees, such as mindfulness workshops, time-management courses, or well-being apps. However, research shows they have little benefit to individuals, with one exception: wellness programs that allow employees to do volunteer work in their community result in employees' greater well-being (Fleming, 2024). For another example, many universities have "service-learning" programs that promote volunteer work. These have been shown to enhance social responsibility among students. Service learning and volunteer work can help emerging adults build social capital, which has many benefits.

How Can You Help Emerging Adults Develop Cultural Competence?

Colleges often require students to take courses in cultural diversity. Does this work? Only about half of students say it increased their capacity to learn from diverse perspectives, and less than a third said that fellow students were respectful when discussing controversial issues from different cultural perspectives. Similarly, participating in co-curricular activities, such as student government or community volunteering does not necessarily lead to cultural competence. In fact, it can lead to strengthened biases if one only participates with one's own "tribe." So, what approaches are successful? Cultural competence can increase through immersion in other cultures, becoming friends with diverse others, and learning about the "good" aspects of other cultures (Lemmer & Wagner, 2015). Reading and watching documentaries about people from other cultures, followed by reflection and discussion, can increase empathy, theory of mind, and multicultural awareness.

Chapter Summary

Developmental tasks that emerging adults, ages 19–25, should be pursuing include self-sufficiency and identity exploration. Their emotion regulation is already fairly mature, so it shows little change, but there are large individual differences between emerging adults in their ability to regulate their emotions. Serious mental health disorders often begin during emerging adulthood. Even though emerging adults are no longer children, they continue to benefit from secure attachment.

Romance is a key developmental task of emerging adulthood. Romantic partners can function like an attachment relationship, providing feelings of security and comfort. Insecure adults are less likely to have satisfying relationships. Identity formation is also a key developmental task in emerging adulthood. Self-narratives help young adults form their identities, and emerging adults in low-income or marginalized communities may use counternarratives to shape their identities.

Emerging adults who are prosocial have advantages because of their strong relationships and social networks, greater mental health, and favorable preparation for jobs and college. On the other hand, antisocial emerging adults tend to experience many problems.

Suggested Readings

Arnett, J. J. (2014). *Emerging adulthood: The winding road from the late teens through the twenties*. Oxford University Press.

Steinberg, L. (2023). *You and your adult child: How to grow together in challenging times*. Simon & Schuster.

References

Ablaza, C., Kabátek, J., & Perales, F. (2022). Are sibship characteristics predictive of same sex marriage? An examination of fraternal birth order and female fecundity effects in population-level administrative data from the Netherlands. *The Journal of Sex Research, 59*(6), 671–683.

Arnett, J. (2015). *Emerging adulthood*. (2nd ed.). Oxford University Press.

Atwell, M. (2023). *The role of social and emotional learning in future workforce readiness*. Penn State Edna Bennett Pierce Prevention Research Center.

Bailey, J. M., Vasey, P. L., Diamond, L. M., Breedlove, S. M., Vilain, E., & Epprecht, M. (2016). Sexual orientation, controversy, and science. *Psychological Science in the Public Interest, 17*(2), 45–101.

Engelhardt, C. R., Bartholow, B. D., & Saults, J. S. (2011). Violent and nonviolent video games differentially affect physical aggression for individuals high vs. low in dispositional anger. *Aggressive Behavior, 37*(6), 539–546.

Fleming, W. J. (2024). Employee well-being outcomes from individual-level mental health interventions: Cross-sectional evidence from the United Kingdom. *Industrial Relations Journal, 55*(2), 162–182.

Gómez-López, M., Viejo, C., & Ortega-Ruiz, R. (2019). Well-being and romantic relationships: A systematic review in adolescence and emerging adulthood. *International Journal of Environmental Research and Public Health, 16*(13), 2415–2446.

Gonzalez Avilés, T., Finn, C. & Neyer, F.J. (2021). Patterns of romantic relationship experiences and psychosocial adjustment From adolescence to young adulthood. *Journal of Youth and Adolescence, 50*(3), 550–562.

Goodwin, G. P. (2015). Moral character in person perception. *Current Directions in Psychological Science, 24*(1), 38–44. https://doi.org/10.1177/0963721414550709

Haas, B. (2019). Enhancing the intercultural competence of college students: A consideration of applied teaching techniques. *International Journal of Multicultural Education, 21*(2), 81–96.

Kessler, R., Berglund, P., Demler, O., Jin, R., Merikangas, K., & Walters, E. (2005). Lifetime prevalence and age-of-onset distributions of DSM-IV disorders in the National Comorbidity Survey Replication. *Archives of General Psychiatry, 62*(6), 593–602.

Kross, E., Berman, M.G., Mischel, W., Smith, E.E., & Wager, T.D. (2011). Social rejection shares somatosensory representations with physical pain. *Proceedings of the National Academy of Sciences, 108*(15), 6270–6275.

Lemmer, G., & Wagner, U. (2015). Can we really reduce ethnic prejudice outside the lab? A meta-analysis of direct and indirect contact interventions. *European Journal of Social Psychology, 45*(2), 152–168.

Loeb, E.L., Kansky, J., Tan, J.S., Costello, M.A., & Allen, J.P. (2021), Perceived psychological control in early adolescence predicts lower levels of adaptation into mid-adulthood. *Child Development, 92*(2): e158–e172.

Nelson, S. K., Layous, K., Cole, S. W., & Lyubomirsky, S. (2016). Do unto others or treat yourself? The effects of prosocial and self-focused behavior on psychological flourishing. *Emotion, 16*(6), 850–861.

Thomas, A. G., Jonason, P. K., Blackburn, J. D., Kennair, L. E. O., Lowe, R., Malouff, J., Stewart-Williams, S., Sulikowski, D., & Li, N. P. (2020). Mate preference priorities in the East and West: A cross-cultural test of the mate preference priority model. *Journal of Personality, 88*(3), 606–620. https://doi.org/10.1111/jopy.12514

Turner, K., Lilgendahl, J. P., Syed, M., & McLean, K. C. (2024). Testing exploratory narrative processing as a mechanism of change in identity status processes over 4 years in college-going emerging adults. *Developmental Psychology, 60*(1), 59–74.

U.S. Surgeon General. (2023). *Our epidemic of loneliness and isolation: The U.S. surgeon general's advisory on the healing effects of social connection and community.* Author.

Waldinger, R. J., & Schulz, M. S. (2016). The long reach of nurturing family environments: Links with midlife emotion-regulatory styles and late-life security in intimate relationships. *Psychological Science, 27*(11), 1443–1450.

Xu, Y., Norton, S., & Rahman, Q. (2019). Early life conditions and adolescent sexual orientation: A prospective birth cohort study. *Developmental Psychology, 55*(6), 1226–1243.

Chapter 7

Theories of Social and Emotional Competence Development

In her sixth grade classroom, Lily was working on math problems using tiles. She became frustrated and asked the girl next to her to "just give me the answers." The other girl said, "I don't think I should do that." Lily then angrily swept all the tiles onto the floor, stomped to her desk, and slammed herself into it. Later, in afterschool art studio, Lily was in a mixed age group activity for fourth to eighth grade girls. The group is designed to build social skills. The girls were hammering nails into a wooden frame so that they could weave yarn on it to make a mosaic. Lily was meticulously hammering in the nails when one went askew. Lily threw her hammer down and began sobbing. An adult said, "Would you like me to help you?" Lily, yelled, "I don't want help!! I want to be able to do it myself!" Lily refused to be consoled or helped with her project.

Why does Lily behave the way she does? How could you help her to behave in a way that allows her to function in school and social groups without being rejected by the other children?

Scientists use theories to answer questions like these. Theories help us to explain and predict how children develop. While every child, and their context, is unique, there are general principles that apply to most people. Theories are a way to organize those principles. Theories focus on age trends (e.g., how is a typical 2-year-old different from a typical 8- or 16-year-old?), as well as on individual and group differences (e.g., why are some 8-year-olds irritable and anxious but others are not?). Since the early 1900s, scientists have conducted careful research studies to test the theories.

Why do you need to know about theories? Because you operate on your personal implicit theories or set of beliefs every time you interact with others. You might have an implicit theory that children need to be free in order to develop optimally; or you might believe that they should be carefully guided, perhaps with rewards and punishments. You might believe that people are most interested in seeking maximum benefits for themselves even if it hurts others; or you might believe that people are concerned with others and willing to help. Your personal theories will influence the way that you engage with children.

DOI: 10.4324/9781003046455-7

It is important to check your implicit theories against theories that have been formally researched. This will help make your personal theories clearer to you, and possibly challenge the accuracy of some. This will also give you insight into children's behavior and help you make good decisions about how to promote children's well-being. In doing so, you will become a better provider of services to your patients, students, and clients.

In this chapter, we will discuss major theories that have stood the test of time for explaining and predicting development from infancy to emerging adulthood – Attachment Theory, Sociocultural Theory, Behaviorism, Social-Cognitive Theory, Self-Determination Theory (SDT) – and the Thriving with Social Purpose (TSP) framework that pulls them together.

Attachment Theory

Attachment Theory asserts that children are born with an innate need for attachment. How adults meet those needs influences children's social–emotional development. In Chapters 3–6, we discussed the remarkably broad effects of secure (vs. insecure) attachment on children's healthy social–emotional development. In later chapters, you will learn that repairing insecure attachment is a primary task of therapists. What does theory say about why attachment is so important?

Through attachment relationships, children create a mental model of themselves and others. These models are expectations, based on memories of how others (typically parents) have interacted with them. Secure children have models of *themselves* as valuable and worthy of being loved and of *others* as caring, responsive, and trustworthy. Insecure children have internal models of themselves as unworthy and others as hostile, inconsistent, and untrustworthy. These models are created through thousands of daily interactions with attachment figures (AFs)s. They are not conscious, which is why they are difficult to change. Children then behave in ways that confirm their internal models, like a self-fulfilling prophecy. For example, a child who expects you to be hostile (due to a history of harsh, critical parents, and insecure attachment) will behave in ways that draw hostility from you, which then confirms their expectation. Part of psychotherapy is to try to change these models and accompanying behaviors that work against children's (or adult's) own well-being.

Even if you are not an actual AF, you can still provide security to youth through a healthy, positive relationship. For example, teachers can be secure attachment-like figures to their students. If you work with insecure children, you will need to be aware of their models of themselves and others, try to counter their models, and rebuild a better model. Feeling secure in a relationship promotes emotional competence.

Sociocultural Theory

Sociocultural Theory (Vygotsky, 1978) asserts that children's development is driven by social interaction. Children grow into the social, emotional, and cultural life of those around them. They grow up inside others' scripts. They do this through *scaffolding* (also called guidance or apprenticeship) where an expert, or more-competent other, supports a child's learning (Smagorinsky, 2018). The expert (typically an adult or older child) breaks the skill into small units the child can perform and guides the child's performance to a higher level. Initially, the child might just observe the expert. Next, the expert does most of the work while guiding the child to help a little. As the child becomes more competent, the expert does less and gives more responsibility for the skill to the child, who grows in expertise. The expert may still need to give hints and reminders, until at last the child is independently competent. For example, in Chapter 3, you learned that adults need to *co-regulate* (i.e., scaffold) toddlers' emotions. Through such scaffolding, children gradually learn to regulate their own emotions. Even older adolescents might need occasional scaffolding with big emotions. For example, a coach might remind an athlete to count to 10 before talking to the referee. Whether a skill is learned quickly, or takes decades to learn, the same mechanism applies. Expecting children to learn complex skills on their own often does not work as well as scaffolding.

Ideally, scaffolding occurs in the child's *zone of proximal development (ZPD)*. This is the level of competence *between*: (1) what a child can do alone and (2) what he or she can do only with substantial help. For example, imagine an older brother is angry that his younger brother took a toy, and hits him. Scaffolding in the zone of proximal development might look like this at different ages:

- Age 2: "Oh no! Don't hit him; you'll hurt him. See he's crying now. Give him this other toy instead."
- Age 5: "You know we don't hit! It hurts others. What can you do instead?"
- Age 10: "No snatching or hitting! I expect you two to work out a compromise!"

The younger the child, the more you do the work in managing the conflict constructively, but you turn over greater responsibility to the child as his ZPD for coping with anger and resolving conflict grows. That growth is a result of your scaffolding such conflicts over and over across years. Without scaffolding, children may experience failure, but with a little help they can be successful. Over time, you should gradually withdraw scaffolding so that children are always in their ZPD. But, keep in mind that the ZPD is a moving target, always changing. It takes attention on your part to continually adjust your scaffolding. Day-to-day scaffolding interactions are the root of social and emotional competence.

A key concept of sociocultural theory is *private speech* (also inner speech or self-talk), which refers to talking to oneself out loud, partially out loud, or silently in one's mind (Flanagan & Symonds, 2022). Private speech helps us guide ourselves when doing something hard in our ZPD. It becomes more internal, and less "out loud" from preschool through the school years. That means young children use it more than adults, but even adults use private speech during problem-solving – such as talking to yourself while trying put together mail-order furniture, or just before you enter a therapy group that you know will be challenging. You may notice children use speech to regulate their emotions, such as distracting themselves in order to avoid becoming angry (Flanagan & Symonds, 2022).

Behaviorism and Social Cognitive Theory

Behaviorism

Behaviorism, also called "learning theory," asserts that humans learn behavior from consequences in the environment (Skinner, 1972). Consequences that increase the probability that you will produce a certain response are called "reinforcement." For example, if a teacher praises students when they give responses in class, the praised students will probably continue giving responses in class. Praise works as a reinforcement. However, some students don't like attention in class; for them, being praised might not increase responses and might even decrease them. What different people find reinforcing can vary. You can *unlearn* behavior by repeatedly giving responses that do not get reinforced, such as if a teacher quit praising students for giving responses in class.

The environment (including other people) shapes your behavior through reinforcement or punishment. Reinforcement could be a smile from someone, a treat, money, or other reward. Punishment decreases behavior. This could be a spanking, time out, being yelled at, or getting fired. A key concept to remember is that *reinforcement and punishment are defined by their outcomes*. That is, if you intend to reduce a teenager's misbehavior by threatening punishment, but the misbehavior does not decrease, then the threat is not actually working as a punishment. The same is true for reinforcement. If you intend to increase good behavior by offering a reward, but good behavior does not increase, then the reward is not actually working as reinforcement.

Two common mistakes people make when using behaviorism is: (1) not reinforcing behaviors that should be reinforced and (2) reinforcing the wrong behaviors. For example, imagine that a child who hates reading misbehaves during his reading class. As "punishment," the teacher sends him to the principal's office, where he gets to escape reading, have a juice box, and play on an iPad. This is not likely to reduce his misbehavior during reading class.

What do you do if a child doesn't ever do what you want? You can't reinforce behavior that doesn't occur. One solution is to "shape" approximations toward the behavior (Gover et al., 2023). This means you reinforce behavior that is close to, or in the direction of, what you want. Over time, you reinforce behavior that gets closer and closer to the target behavior. Psychologists use shaping very carefully by setting clear goals, consistently reinforcing behavior in increments, giving immediate feedback, and providing adequate time for growth.

To make behaviorism work, you must know what the person finds reinforcing. You can't assume that what you find reinforcing will be just as reinforcing to someone else. One of us worked at a high-school carnival. At each booth, if the teenagers won a game, they got to choose a prize of either a dollar or a piece of penny candy. Adults assumed they'd want the dollars. Guess which the teenagers preferred? If you guessed penny candy, you are right. At the end of the event, the candy was gone, but dollar bills were left over.

Behaviorism works. We can change our own, others, and even our dog's behavior using behaviorism. We are all constantly influenced by the pattern of reinforcement and punishment operating in our lives. One of the most famous behaviorist psychologists, Skinner (1972), argued that we should try to make ourselves aware of the reinforcers that influence us, so that we are not controlled without awareness, and that we should use reinforcement to better others' condition, such as helping antisocial youth stay out of prison. He thought we could create utopia by using behaviorism wisely. He wrote a book about it called *Walden Two* that described a utopian society based on behaviorist principles, especially reinforcement. In the book, children were raised communally, there was gender equality, and everyone was happy.

However, there are two cautions about behaviorism. First, many psychologists, including behaviorists, are opposed to punishment, believing that we should primarily focus on reinforcement. Skinner argued that it is better to reinforce the behavior you want rather than punish the behavior you do not want. While punishment might sometimes reduce behavior, it often doesn't work as intended; for example, punishment can influence people to attempt to escape the punishment rather than change their behavior. In addition: (1) punishment does not teach replacement behavior, which is not helpful when the underlying problem is lack of skill or not knowing what the expectations are, (2) children do not internalize principles of good behavior from punishment, and (3) punishment often devolves into power assertive discipline with all the serious costs of power assertive discipline discussed in Chapter 4.

Second, while material rewards do work in the short-term, they can undermine motivation in the long-term. That is, if you give children treats, money, or other rewards for something, such as sitting quietly during church, they are less likely to internalize the value of sitting quietly. How does this happen? When children are offered a reward, they think "I am doing this to get the reward" instead of "I am doing this because it is the right thing to do." (This thought is not necessarily conscious.) Material rewards also train children to ask "what's in it for me?" for behaviors that should simply be expected. Note that this only pertains to tangible, material rewards. If the reward is *social* and subtle (e.g., a nod of approval or praise), then children may think "I am doing this because I choose to." In contrast to material rewards, social rewards do not undermine motivation or short circuit the development of self-control.

Use of material rewards does not have these negative repercussions under two conditions: (1) when they are unexpected, such having an impromptu party to celebrate an achievement and (2) when there is no motivation for the behavior to begin with. You can't undermine motivation that does not exist. For example, some families give treats to toddlers for using the potty if the toddler has no interest in potty-training (but the parents do!).

Most adults use reinforcement and punishment on children, whether intentional or not. It is best not to use it if you want to help children develop internal motivation and self-control. If you feel you must use behaviorism because there is no intrinsic motivation in a child to behave, or behavior is out of control, then you might use it briefly until behavior becomes more appropriate. Then, gradually transition to use of induction instead. If you are working with a group of children, where some, but not all, of the children may need behavior modification, you can use it on the subset who need it. However, generally praise, rather than material rewards, is a powerful enough reinforcer that you do not need material rewards, even for challenging children.

Let's apply these principles to prosocial behavior. Research robustly finds that giving children material rewards for behaving prosocially might increase it in the short-term, but over the long-term, children will engage in less prosocial behavior. However, research also finds that praising children for behaving prosocially results in greater prosocial behavior over time.

Social Cognitive Theory

Imagine you are teaching a group of children to repair a bicycle tire. Two children help each other. You smile and say "Thank you for helping each other. Way to be a team!" As a result, in a few weeks when the class meets again, other children who overheard you may start helping each other. This example illustrates two key points: (1) Children can learn from watching others be reinforced (or punished) without being directly reinforced (or punished) themselves, called *vicarious reinforcement*. (2) Children can learn without immediate behavior change; learning might not be apparent for weeks or years later. These points may seem obvious, but they challenge classic behaviorism which defines "learning" as a "change in behavior." Obviously, you can learn without changing your

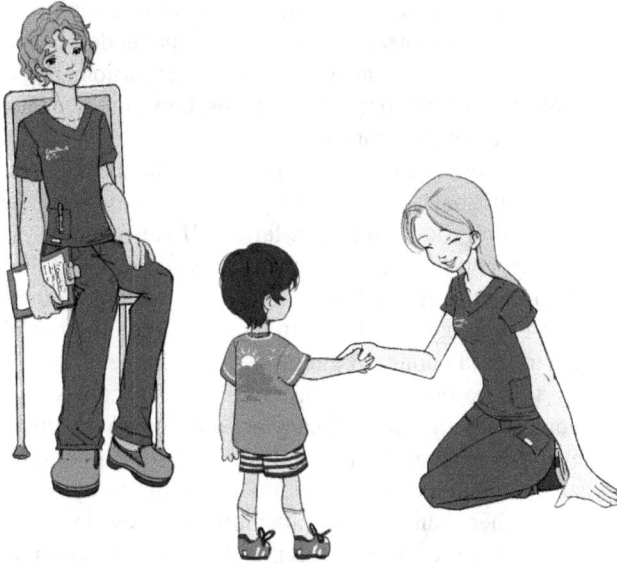

Figure 7.1 According to Sociocultural and Social Cognitive Theories, infants to adults learn through observing competent others.

behavior. This led to a refined version of behaviorism called "social cognitive theory" (see Figure 7.1).

Social cognitive theory asserts that you learn from reinforcement, but also from interaction with others around you and from your beliefs about your ability. Behavior is strongly influenced by your *self-efficacy,* which is your belief that you are capable of accomplishing a specific behavior (Bandura, 1997). For example, if Gerald does not think he is capable of repairing a bicycle tire, even if he sees others being reinforced for working together, Gerald is not likely to attempt bicycle repair. The name of this theory has the word "cognitive" in it because self-efficacy is a cognition – meaning it is related to thinking. One of the authors of this book saw Skinner in old age give a lecture. He pounded the lectern loudly proclaiming that "there is no need to bring cognition into the discussion!" because behavior can be explained by simple reinforcement. He was wrong. Humans are also influenced by the way they think about a situation, including their self-efficacy.

Self-efficacy pertains to specific behaviors. You might have high self-efficacy for making friends, but low self-efficacy for public speaking. Self-efficacy comes from your history of success and failure, but also from witnessing vicarious reinforcement of a model similar to you. Gerald might come to believe he is capable of repairing a bicycle tire if he sees someone quite similar to himself do it. This is why the peer model of therapy you will learn about in Chapter 10 is so useful. Clients learn from interacting with peers who model social–emotional competencies. Self-efficacy can also come from persuasion. For example, a teacher or therapist might point out your strengths, how you used them in a situation, and convince you of your capability.

Self-efficacy is important because it influences whether you take on challenging tasks, set high goals, and improve your skills. This is because it influences the way you think about success or failure. If you attribute your failings to something inside you that can't be changed, you are more likely to give up when faced with challenge or avoid things that are hard. You might think, "I failed because I'm no good at this." In contrast, you might think "I failed because I didn't try hard enough; I am going to try harder." In this case, you are more likely to take on challenging tasks, set high goals, and improve your skills. People with high self-efficacy are more likely to attribute failure to effort, recover faster from failure, and try harder. Professionals can help patients, students, and clients who have low self-efficacy by retraining them to make helpful, rather than harmful, attributions. They do this by helping clients use better strategies and by giving them opportunities for success with feedback to enhance skills. For example, they might help clients who have high self-efficacy for resolving a conflict with aggression, but low self-efficacy for using compromise, work on conflict resolutions skills with supportive feedback.

Let's apply this to prosocial behavior. Children are more likely to become prosocial over time if they are in a setting, such as a classroom, with peers who model prosocial behavior. This even pertains to learning from media. Youth who play prosocial videogames are more likely to develop empathy and prosocial behavior.

Unfortunately, the same influences occur for antisocial behavior. Research robustly finds that youth who are exposed to aggressive models in movies and videogames become desensitized to aggression, increase in aggression, and decrease in sympathy and prosocial behavior (Coyne et al., 2018; Han & Carlo, 2021). The more exposure to antisocial models in media that you experience, the more your own attitudes align with antisocial behavior because your moral orientation toward helping others in need will erode. The "general aggression model" (GAM) is often used to explain aggression and incorporates social cognitive theory. According to the GAM, in the instant that a person may choose to be aggressive or prosocial, a trigger in the setting interacts with the person's "action tendencies" that prepare them to be more or less aggressive, leading toward thoughts and emotions that drive aggressive behavior (Anderson & Bushman, 2018). What might lead to aggressive action tendencies? Aggressive models, reinforcement for aggression, desensitization toward aggression, and low empathy for others.

Self-Determination Theory (SDT)

According to SDT, humans are driven by an internal need to grow (Ryan & Deci, 2020). In contrast to behaviorism, it focuses on our *inner* life. SDT asserts that humans have three basic psychological needs: autonomy (or self-determination), belongingness, and competence. Feeling competent is part of self-efficacy, which we've already discussed. We'll focus on belonging and autonomy here.

Belongingness refers to feeling like you are accepted and cared about in your group. It is about having meaningful relationships. Healthy relationships are the foundation of social–emotional well-being. You will learn in Chapters 10 and 11 that much of the work of therapists is to help their clients establish healthier relationships. Professionals who form warm, trusting relationships, are empathic, and are non-judgmental are more likely to promote better and more sustained outcomes and increased motivation to adhere to treatment plans among their clients.

Autonomy refers to feeling like you have control over what you do. You pursue things with greater motivation if you feel like you have chosen them. Of course, free choice is not always possible or ideal. For example, U.S. states have compulsory education laws, and traffic lights tell you whether to go or stop. Guidance and structure are often helpful. Nevertheless, some sense of choice over your action is important.

Teachers who foster autonomy by giving students choice over learning activities (e.g., which book to read or which science project to pursue) promote greater engagement and learning in their students. Therapists can foster autonomy by encouraging clients to make their own choices, explore their values, and set goals so that they feel empowered to control their therapeutic course. Healthcare professionals can foster autonomy by helping patients make decisions and set their own goals (perhaps with scaffolding). For example, a physical therapist might offer choices in exercises and give feedback on improvements to a patient recovering from an injury.

In the section on behaviorism above, we discussed how material rewards undermine motivation in the long-term. This is partly because they conflict with autonomy. Rewards can feel overly controlling or manipulative to youth and adults. We also discussed the serious costs of punishment. Punishment, like material rewards, also conflicts with autonomy. Punishment is particularly negative because it also undermines belongingness and makes youth feel angry and rejected. This results in less, not more, motivation to obey the disciplinarian. Recall from Chapter 4 that power assertive discipline results in *less* obedience in the long-term. This is ironic because adults punish children in order to increase obedience. Yet, a large meta-analysis of 85 studies with thousands of participants across cultures found that when adults give youth autonomy, the youth are more prosocial (Donald et al., 2021). In contrast, when adults use more control, youth display more antisocial behavior, rebellion, anger, and rejection of the adult's values. How did adults give youth autonomy? They used inductive discipline and provided choice. What kind of control did the adults use? They used controlling language (e.g., you must do this) and rewards (or bribes) to manipulate children's behavior.

Putting the Theories Together: The Thriving through Social Purpose (TSP) Framework

Each of these major theories is supported by research, yet each is incomplete by itself. There currently is no single grand theory that adequately unifies them. However, the TSP framework brings them together to help us understand how children can thrive (Ford & Smith, 2007). According to the TSP framework, thriving is the result of having positive goals, high self-efficacy, and positive emotions working together constructively. Although individuals have unique goals, there are core goals shared by most people. These are belongingness, autonomy, competence, and being prosocial toward others (Bergin, 2019; Ryan & Deci, 2020). Emotions interact with self-efficacy to influence whether you pursue goals because emotions focus attention and activate behavior. According to TSP, when individuals' goals involve concern for others and individuals have self-efficacy that they can achieve those goals (in a context with scaffolding to become competent), they will come to feel positive emotions through healthy relationships. When these qualities are integrated, they amplify social–emotional well-being. Thus, contexts that combine prosocial goals, positive emotions, secure relationships, and self-efficacy will be powerful in promoting optimal development in infants to emerging adults. Social–emotional well-being then leads to personal optimism and trust in others, which in turn provides a deep motivational well as individuals thrive.

Chapter Summary

Attachment Theory asserts that children are born with an innate need for attachment. How adults meet attachment needs influences children's social–emotional development. Sociocultural Theory asserts that children learn through guidance from more competent others. Children learn by actively doing while being scaffolded by more competent others, like adults or older children. Social Cognitive Theory asserts that children learn through reinforcement (as in classic Behaviorism) but also learn through observation. Children then form beliefs about themselves and their capabilities, including self-efficacy. Self-determination Theory asserts that humans are motivated by feelings of autonomy, belonging, and competence. No single theory can explain everything about children's social–emotional development, but these theories explain enough to help us create better environments for children and to guide the practice of professionals who work with infants to emerging adults.

In the following chapters, you will see how professionals can help children develop greater social–emotional competence. You'll notice that some strategies keep coming up again and again across different professions and roles because, as these theories highlight, they are foundational. The common strategies include: (1) foster secure attachment, (2) use inductive discipline, especially other-oriented induction, (3) praise prosocial behavior, (4) directly coach constructive coping strategies, (5) talk about emotions to promote recognizing and understanding emotions, and (6) create a positive emotional climate.

References

Anderson, C.A. and Bushman, B.J. (2018), Media violence and the General Aggression Model. *Journal of Social Issues, 74*(2), 386–413.

Bandura, A. (1997). *Self-efficacy: The exercise of control.* Freeman.

Bergin, C. (2019). Prosocial goals in the classroom. In M. H. Jones (Ed.), *Social goals in the classroom: Findings on student motivation and peer relations* (pp. 93–110). Routledge.

Coyne, S. M., Warburton, W., Essig, L. W., & Stockdale, L. (2018). Violent video games, externalizing behavior, and prosocial behavior: A five-year longitudinal study during adolescence. *Developmental Psychology, 54*(10), 1868–1880.

Donald, J. N., Bradshaw, E. L., Conigrave, J. H., Parker, P. D., Byatt, L. L., Noetel, M., & Ryan, R. M. (2021). Paths to the light and dark sides of human nature: A meta-analytic review of the prosocial benefits of autonomy and the antisocial costs of control. *Psychological Bulletin, 147*(9), 921–946.

Flanagan, R., & Symonds, J. (2022). Children's self-talk in naturalistic classroom settings in middle childhood: A systematic review. *Educational Research Review, 35*, 100432.

Ford, M., & Smith, P. (2007). Thriving with social purpose: An integrative approach to the development of optimal human functioning. *Educational Psychologist, 42*(3), 153–171.

Gover, H. C., Hanley, G. P., Ruppel, K. W., Landa, R. K., & Marcus, J. (2023). Prioritizing choice and assent in the assessment and treatment of food selectivity. *International Journal of Developmental Disabilities, 69*(1), 53–65.

Han, Y., & Carlo, G. (2021). The links between religiousness and prosocial behaviors in early adulthood: The mediating roles of media exposure preferences and empathic tendencies. *Journal of Moral Education, 50*(4), 419–435.

Ryan, R. M., & Deci, E. L. (2020). Intrinsic and extrinsic motivation from a self-determination theory perspective: Definitions, theory, practices, and future directions. *Contemporary Educational Psychology, 61*, 101860.

Skinner, B. F. (1972). *Cumulative record: A selection of papers* (3rd ed.). Appleton-Century-Crofts.

Smagorinsky, P. (2018). Deconflating the ZPD and instructional scaffolding: Retranslating and reconceiving the zone of proximal development as the zone of next development. *Learning, Culture and Social Interaction, 16*, 70–75.

Vygotsky, L. S. (1978). *Mind in society: The development of higher psychological processes*. Harvard University Press.

Chapter 8

Applying Social and Emotional Competence in the Allied Health Fields

Penny has been a Child Life Specialist for 6 years. She works in a hospital with children from birth to 3 months, focusing on newly formed families and premature babies. Some premature babies stay in the hospital beyond 3 months. Families come to rely on her for emotional support through this major life change and to help them learn to care for a fragile baby when they are ready to take the baby home. Some families return for a reunion when the baby is 1 year old. The hospital staff really enjoy these reunions because they like to see that fragile babies they cared for are now growing.

Penny is an allied health professional. Two fields that touch almost all children are medicine and education. Most children are involved with medicine from the time before they are born through prenatal care, then at birth, followed by well-baby care at the doctors' office. Well-baby care involves regular doctor visits – at 1 month, 2 months, 4 months, 6 months, 9 months, 12 months, 15 months, 18 months, and 2 years – where the baby is measured for growth, checked for developmental milestones, and given immunizations. After early childhood, most children will only encounter the medical field for immunizations or annual physical exams unless they have an injury or illness (e.g., ear infection). However, some children may have long-term or frequent physical and medical needs that require support from allied health professionals. Common long-term conditions among children include asthma, ADHD, chronic ear infections, cystic fibrosis, autism, epilepsy, cerebral palsy, obesity, and diabetes.

Who Is an Allied Health Professional?

The most common allied health professionals you may be aware of are doctors, nurses, and dentists. Doctors who specialize in medical care for children are called pediatricians, and those who specialize in newborns are neonatologists. (Neonates are babies less than a month old.) Nurses and dentists who specialize in children are called pediatric nurses and pediatric dentists, respectively. Yet, there are many other kinds of professionals who work in the health field with infants to emerging adults. These include physical therapists, pharmacists,

DOI: 10.4324/9781003046455-8

occupational therapists, dental hygienists, dieticians, audiologists, speech pathologists, medical technicians, and many more. Within each field, there may be different roles. For example, medical technicians might be radiologic technicians (someone who administers sonographs), lab technicians (someone who analyzes samples of body fluids), emergency medical technicians (EMTs; someone who rides ambulances to tend to injured people at the scene of emergencies), and many more kinds of technicians. New roles are constantly emerging as new medical advances are made. (You can view a list of allied health professions at the U.S. National Institute of Health or at the U.K. National Health Service.)

It is not clear which professionals are included in the term "allied health." A commission in 1980 took six pages to discuss what the term should include! We will use the much shorter U.S. National Institute of Health (NIH) definition of allied health: *all health personnel working toward the common goal of providing the best possible service in patient care and health promotion.* They intentionally leave the term a little vague. As a result, different organizations have somewhat different definitions. The NIH definition is intended to acknowledge that it often takes a team of people with different expertise to help individuals struggling with physical challenges or illnesses.

Allied health professionals may work in different kinds of settings, such as directly with patients, in labs (e.g., testing blood samples), or in administrative and community work (e.g., health promotion). Direct patient work may be in a hospital, doctor's office, clinic, home, or other setting. For example, some EMTs and paramedics are based in fire stations and minister to patients in their homes or on the street. Other allied health professionals work in schools, such as Aaryn, described in Case Study Box 8.1.

Box 8.1   Occupational Therapist Case Study

Aaryn is an occupational therapist. This means she helps people with limitations learn functional skills to deal with daily life. Aaryn works in a hospital and in two middle schools. At the hospital, she helps children who have just had leg surgery. When they are ready to leave the hospital to go home, she teaches them how to get in and out of a car safely and go up the step into their house. At the schools, she helps children with Down Syndrome learn to do basic tasks at school, such as how to wash their hands. Without training, the children quickly dip one hand in water, then shake it off. She teaches them to use both hands and rub them together with soap before rinsing. The goal of this functional skill is that the children will be safe from transmitting or catching illnesses in school.

Some allied health professionals may work in behavioral health care, such as substance misuse treatment. They help patients with the process of recovery, including how to handle negative emotions without using substances. They may also help a person who is physically addicted to substances such as alcohol or opioids handle withdrawal through supervised use of medications. Thus, there are many kinds of allied health professionals.

How Do You Become an Allied Health Professional?

While it is not entirely clear what kinds of workers can be called an allied health professional, NIH does require that workers with this title meet three requirements: (1) work in a health-specific industry (2) have formal, advanced training in healthcare, and (3) work in a field that requires licensure for the workers and accreditation for educational settings that train the workers. The training for different kinds of allied health professionals varies widely. At the extremely advanced level, specialized physicians may spend 12 years after high school in rigorous schooling, such as a pediatric cardiologist, and receive a specialized medical doctoral degree. At the entry level, a lab assistant might just need 1 or 2 years of training and a certificate. Many assistant positions, such as a respiratory assistant who works with children with asthma, may require a 2-year associate's degree, but assistant positions may also require a bachelor's or master's degree (including respiratory assistants) to advance their career and competencies. Some assistant positions, such as physician's assistant, require master's degrees, clinical experience with supervision, and then passing a certification exam.

How Do Allied Health Professionals Promote Social–Emotional Competence in Children and Youth?

Recall that emotional competence refers to being able to regulate your own emotions and accurately read others' emotions. Social competence refers to being more prosocial, less antisocial, and able to interact effectively with others. Having self-control, a healthy sense of self, and well-adjusted personality are the result of social–emotional competencies. So, how do allied health professionals help children develop these competencies?

First, it is important that professionals display social–emotional competence themselves. This is particularly important given that allied health professionals work with children during stressful and emotional times in their lives. Children may be in pain or frightened. Professionals can increase their own social–emotional competence and their understanding of children by learning about the factors that support children's social–emotional development – such as reading books like this one!

Professionals can also increase their own social–emotional competence by having "practice experiences" integrated into their training (Nagarajan &

McAllister, 2015). For example, as physicians train, they should spend time with child patients. However, some practice experiences are more effective than others. Some ways to improve effectiveness of practice experiences include:

- Have trainees write reflections on their experience and then discuss it with others.
- Have a supervising mentor guide trainees and model behavior.
- Include real-life case studies during training. Have experienced professionals share real conundrums, confrontations, and challenges for trainees to discuss and problem solve as a group.
- Have trainees role play being a child patient.

Such training should continue as pre-professionals begin working with real patients, including continued reflection to identify their strengths and weaknesses. Such activities help professionals improve their own social–emotional competence and become more effective at promoting and protecting the social–emotional competence of their child patients.

Second, like Penny, professionals need to understand how to promote social–emotional competence of children in their care. Allied health professionals should not only be concerned with the physical health of children and youth, but also the social–emotional well-being of the whole child. Social–emotional well-being helps with healing, pain management, immune responses, and mental health in patients and their families.

An interesting example of what happens when children's social–emotional needs are ignored by health professionals occurred in hospital newborn nurseries. Babies used to routinely be separated from their mothers at birth. The nurses fed the babies with bottles, and mothers could only "visit" with their babies for a brief time. There was a pervasive myth that this was *best* for the babies. Nurses and doctors were not adequately aware of babies' social needs. Two pediatricians, Dr. Klaus and Dr. Kennell, noticed that this was *not best*, and advocated that mothers and their infants be kept together (Klein et al., 2018). They said that babies should be breastfed soon after birth so that they could bond with their mother. Thanks to their advocacy, most hospitals now have 24-hour "rooming in" so that babies and mothers are kept together, fathers are present at deliveries, and siblings can visit the baby. This pattern of mother–baby care supports stronger attachment, better breastfeeding, improved sleep quality, reduced infant crying, and reduced postpartum depression in mothers. Klaus and Kennell also advocated that grieving parents who lost a baby at birth should be able to hold their newborn, and they recommended that doulas be in hospitals. Their work has helped hospitals become more sensitive to the social–emotional needs of babies and their mothers. Let's revisit Penny's experience as a child life specialist in Box 8.2.

Box 8.2   Interview of a Child Life Specialist

Penny believes babies should be in sync with and attach to others, especially their parents. She always thinks about social–emotional concepts while working with premature babies and their families. She may suggest the parents take the baby for a stroll, or she may teach the parents, especially young parents, basic caretaking behaviors.

Can you give an example of how you have supported attachment?

Sometimes, I have to make rules in order for all the families to get along. For instance, one mother sang to her baby at feeding time. The mother also read books to her baby, rocked her baby, and talked to her baby. I knew these were all great behaviors for promoting the baby's social–emotional well-being. However, other families in the neonatal room were upset because they felt the noise was disruptive and not good for their babies who were ill. So, I asked the mother who was giving her baby such great stimulation to do it according to a schedule. This rule allowed all families in the neonatal unit to get along and respect each other. I really admired that mom for enhancing her baby's development. This type of stimulation is great for all children, especially premature babies. It definitely helps with social–emotional competence.

Why is it important for child life specialists to understand social–emotional development?

It is important because the whole family is experiencing a stressful event that is new to them. Sometimes, adult family members need social–emotional coaching. All professionals in the field of allied health should know concepts of social–emotional development. New professionals should listen to their mentor and be observant. They should be socially and emotionally competent so that they can understand and communicate with other people and be sensitive to the fact that birth is a stressful time for babies and families. I first learned about social–emotional development in college and then continued to learn more with additional schooling and a certification internship.

Figure 8.1 shows a model to help professionals think about how to support children's social–emotional development. At the base of the pyramid is a well-educated workforce that knows how to use evidence-based practices.

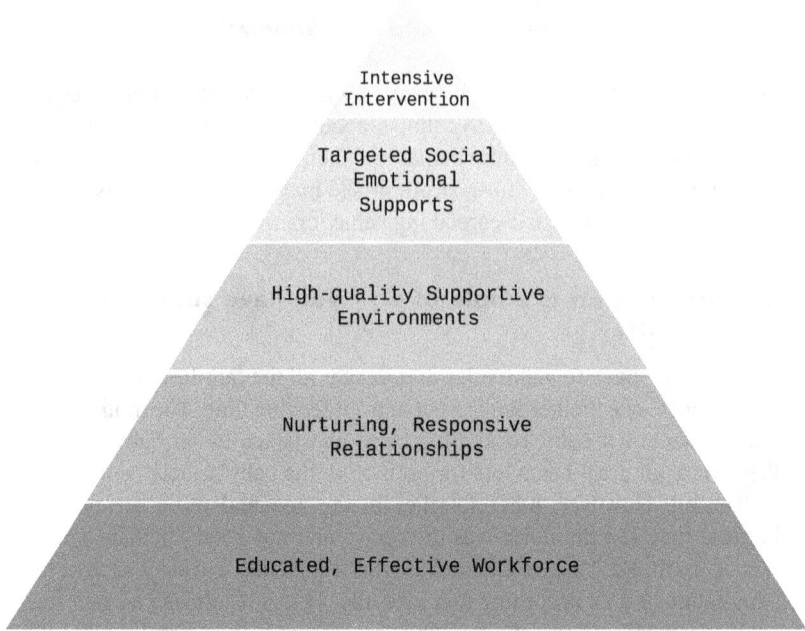

Figure 8.1 Allied health professionals can provide support for patients' social–emotional competencies in multiple ways.

Source: The Center on the Social and Emotional Foundations of Early Learning; Biddle (2021).

Next, a primary way that allied health professionals support children's social–emotional development is to create a safe and nurturing environment. This entails the next two levels of the pyramid. Professionals form supportive, responsive relationships with children. They provide services in an environment that is friendly and welcoming, such as child-sized furniture, play spaces, and calming colors on the walls in rooms for young children. We'll skip the top rung because allied health professionals are not likely to provide intensive intervention for behavior challenges; such work is usually the role of mental health professionals (see Chapters 10 and 11). So, let's discuss targeted social–emotional supports next.

Promoting Emotional Competence

Allied health professionals can promote patients' emotional competence by using the evidence-based practices discussed in Chapters 3–6 to provide supportive environments. These practices include:

1. Provide consistent, predictable care so that children feel secure and are not startled by anything unexpected. Professionals should remain calm, gentle, and highly responsive to children.
2. Give children who are wary gradual exposure to a new situation. Give them as much control as possible. Try to adjust the environment to fit with what makes the child comfortable as the child warms up to the situation (see section on shy children in Chapter 4).
3. Talk with children to help them identify and label their emotions. Children who can label their feelings can better manage the feelings. Validate their feelings and provide reassurance. Some hospitals use play or art therapy to help children express their emotions.

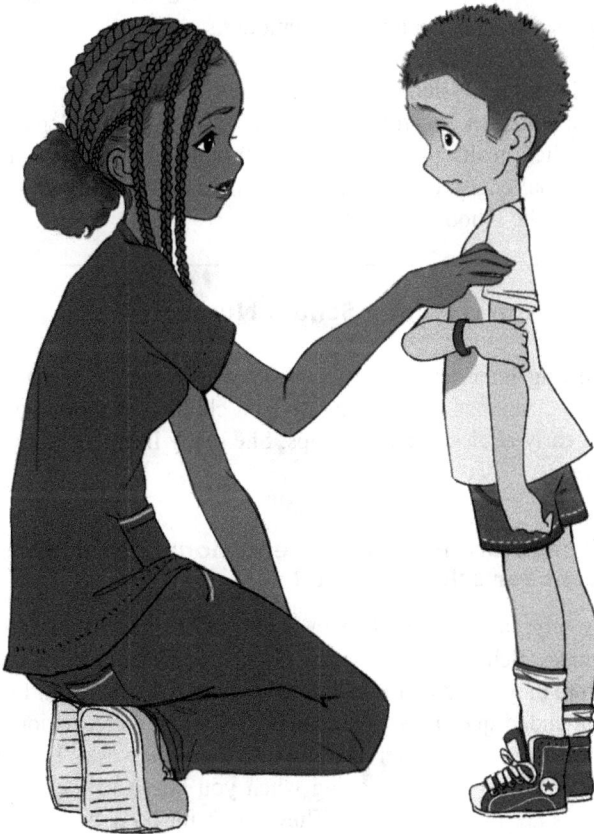

Figure 8.2 Allied health professionals can help children manage emotionally challenging situations.

4. Co-regulate children who have not yet learned to control their emotions. See Chapter 3 for how to soothe and shush an infant. Research finds these techniques are effective in medical settings.

5. Help children use constructive coping strategies (Box 1.1) to reduce stress or cope with big emotions. Don't forget that reappraisal is often (but not always) the best coping strategies for situations the individual cannot control. If a child is not able to cope, advocate for mental health services.

6. Encourage independence by letting children do what they can for themselves. Help children set, monitor, and achieve goals toward managing their health. Celebrate each achievement.

7. Create emotionally upbeat environments, where mostly positive emotions are experienced, but where it is also safe to express authentic, reasonable negative emotions. For example, we have watched pediatricians take a few minutes to play peek-a-boo with a toddler or do a magic trick or tell a corny joke with teenagers to elicit positive emotions.

As Figure 8.2 shows, physicians and other health professionals can help children cope with fear and other negative emotions during health care. School nurses are one type of allied health professional who frequently deal with children who have emotion challenges. Let's see how Felicity deals with the emotions of students in her middle school in Box 8.3.

Box 8.3   Interview of a School Nurse

The following interview is with Felicity who has been a school nurse for 25 years. She has worked mostly with children in the middle childhood and early adolescent age groups. She really likes her work and her workplace.

Why is understanding social–emotional development important for school nurses?

It is very important for children in general, but especially important to school nurses. School nurses have to understand what is going on with a child before they can diagnose the problem and help the child. I ask children open-ended questions to facilitate a two-way conversation. I don't want a "yes" or "no" answer to my questions. I may ask "How are you feeling?" or "What was happening when you began to feel this way?" Most nurses are fairly observant. They watch for body language to give the words a context. They ask the correct type of questions, which are open-ended. These skills make for a good nurse who protects and understands the social–emotional competence of all children.

I learned about children's social–emotional competence when I was in college. Its importance became more vital on the job. I observed and studied colleagues. I even learned from individual, self-guided study of social–emotional competence.

What advice do you have for new school nurses?

Remember that each child is unique. All children have different backgrounds. All have varied and different abilities. Be careful not to negatively judge someone, especially children. Do not judge their parents either. Try to see things from the perspectives of the child, parents, and family system.

Promoting Social Competence

Allied health professionals should work to have positive relationships with parents. Professionals should also support parents in their parenting, such has helping them read or play games with their child while in the clinic or hospital. Penny wanted to support the mother in her neonatal unit who was singing, reading, and talking to her baby because she knows how important this is for secure attachment to develop, so she found a way to support it while also accommodating the other families in the neonatal unit.

Allied health professionals can also facilitate relationships between children in group activities, for example, in a pediatric ward in a hospital or in out-patient services for children with shared conditions. They may organize group games to build children's social–emotional skills (Vallis, 2020). The skills learned from natural interactions during games can carry over to other parts of the children's lives. For instance, teamwork, feedback acceptance, appropriate behavior for wins and losses, setting and meeting goals, and solving problems are all skills that increase social–emotional competence. During group activities, allied health professionals should support prosocial behavior among the children by using the strategies discussed in Chapters 3–6. These include:

1. Praise young patients when they are prosocial, building their sense of identity as a prosocial person.
2. Give them opportunities to practice being prosocial.
3. Use inductive discipline, instead of power assertion, when they misbehave. This promotes prosocial behavior and self-control. See Chapter 4 for how to do this.

4. Scaffold conflict resolution skills of negotiation and compromise, such as turn taking.

Professionals can also implement evidence-based programs. One example is the PATHS (Promoting Alternative Thinking Strategies) program that is designed to reduce aggression and disruptive behavior in children ages 4–11. It can be used in healthcare settings when children have fear, anxiety, or other negative or disruptive emotions. PATHS has lesson plans to teach specific skills through stories, pictures, and puppets. The lessons center on: (1) friendship skills and prosocial behavior, (2) understanding and labeling feelings, (3) exercising self-control in behavior and emotions, and (4) solving social conflicts in a positive manner. In other words, the program uses strategies you learned about in Chapters 3–6. It has been rated as "well-supported by research" from government watchdog agencies such as the federal government's What Works Clearinghouse and the California Evidence-Based Clearinghouse for Child Welfare. Allied health professionals may also select other programs. For example, child life specialists may use a program in a community-based setting for children with cancer. Or, psychiatrists may use one for families with children addicted to drugs or children diagnosed with anxiety. Whichever program is selected, it should be evidence-based (Aarons, 2005), which means there is solid research showing its success with the kinds of families or children that it is intended for, and staff should be trained to use it with fidelity.

As allied health professionals decide how to support children in their care, they may want to ask these questions (Biddle, 2021):

1. Will the professional interact with the child for the short- or long-term or both?
2. What goals does the professional and family have for the child?
3. What community and policy support does the professional have that affects the child's social–emotional competence?
4. Does the professional share the same culture as the child? Does the professional understand the child's culture?

All of these questions will affect the child, the family, and the child's display of social–emotional competence.

Chapter Summary

In summary, there are many kinds of allied health professional roles that work with infants to emerging adults regularly. Therefore, understanding and promoting social–emotional competence in patients is important. Strategies that research suggests will be effective are discussed above.

References

Aarons, G. A. (2005). Measuring provider attitudes toward adoption of evidence-based practice: Considerations of organizational context and individual differences. *Child and Adolescent Psychiatric Clinics of North America, 14*(2), 255–271.

Biddle, K. (2021). Social and emotional learning. In A. Garcia-Nevarez & K. Biddle (Eds.), *Developmentally appropriate curriculum and instruction: pedagogy for knowledge, attitudes, and values* (pp. 145–160). Routledge.

Klein, M. C., Simkin, P., & Young, D. (2018). "Be kind to the mother": A celebration of the life of Marshall Klaus, 1927–2017. *Birth. 45*(1), 3–6.

Nagarajan, S., & McAllister, L. (2015). Integration of practice experiences into the Allied Health Curriculum: Curriculum and pedagogic considerations before, during and after work-integrated learning experiences. *Asia-Pacific Journal of Cooperative Education 16*(4), 279–290.

Vallis, R. (2020). Building social-emotional competence of elementary students through noncompetitive basketball embedded with social skills training. *BU Journal of Graduate Studies in Education 12*(2), 4–7.

Chapter 9

Applying Social and Emotional Competence in Education

Brock was a special education teacher for 11 years. He worked with children who had behavioral challenges. The children would blurt out during class, get into fights, defy teachers, and were failing to learn. They were often suspended from school for aggression. He decided that he needed more training, so he went to graduate school. While there, Brock became committed to doing research on how to help youth with behavior problems. He is now a professor who teaches teachers how to help children replace challenging behaviors and build social skills so they can be successful in school.

In Chapter 8, we said that two fields that touch almost all children are medicine and education. Some children will enter educational settings before kindergarten, referred to as early childhood settings. Almost all children are involved with education because schooling is compulsory in the US. starting around age 5–8 and ending around age 16–19. Other countries have similar requirements. In the US., children in elementary through high school spend more of their time (almost 20%) in school than any other single activity except sleep. Thus, educators have tremendous potential to influence children's social–emotional development. After graduating from compulsory schooling, many emerging adults will continue in education settings such as vocational schooling or university (see Chapter 6).

Who Is an Educator?

An educator is anyone who provides education to others. When people hear the term "educator," most think of teachers who work in preschool through high school (preK-12) settings. Yet, education can take place in other settings, such as vocational training institutions, universities, sports teams, and medical training. In addition, most of the staff who work in preK-12 settings are referred to as educators although they may not teach classes. For example, school counselors, social workers, therapists, and administrators are considered educators in preK-12 schools.

DOI: 10.4324/9781003046455-9

How Do You Become an Educator?

The process of becoming a teacher is a little more demanding the older the children you teach. To become a *preschool teacher*, you need at least an associate's degree or, depending on the state, you may need a credential. To become an *elementary teacher,* you need a bachelor's degree, for which you take courses in child development, teaching methods, classroom management, and educational psychology. You must teach the student under the supervision of a mentor teacher and pass exams such as the Praxis. Then, you must get a certification or license to teach in public schools. The process to become a *secondary teacher* is similar to elementary teachers except that you must have a bachelor's degree (or concentration) in the subject area you will be teaching (e.g., math, social studies). School administrators typically need experience as a teacher, as well as a master's or doctorate (EdD) in educational leadership or administration, and may have to pass license exams. To become a school counselor or school psychologist, you typically need a masters' degree and license or certification which requires passing a test. All educators who work with children must pass criminal background checks to ensure the safety of the children they work with.

Teachers of emerging adults may work in trade schools, colleges, or universities. They are typically called an instructor or professor in the U.S. (or called "lecturers" in other countries). To become an instructor in a *trade school,* you need work experience and a certificate or license in your field, which tends to be more important than formal education. However, to become an instructor in a *community college* you usually must have at least a master's degree. To become a professor at a *university* you typically need a doctorate (PhD) which is the highest level of school degrees. Earning a PhD usually takes 3–6 years of advanced coursework after a master's degree. At most universities, professors are expected to teach *and* generate new knowledge through ongoing research and publications.

How Do Educators Promote Social–Emotional Competence in Children and Youth?

There has been a 50-year trend toward more disruptive behavior and mental health challenges in K-12 students. From 2000 to 2020, verbal abuse and disrespect toward teachers increased nationally (Irwin et al. 2022). This was prior to COVID-19; after the pandemic, there was an additional sharp increase in behavioral challenges. This pattern of misbehavior suggests that teachers need more tools for helping students develop social–emotional competencies. Fortunately, research finds that teachers can make a difference in their students' social–emotional competencies that is as big as or bigger than in their academic learning. We'll discuss key strategies that research suggests work.

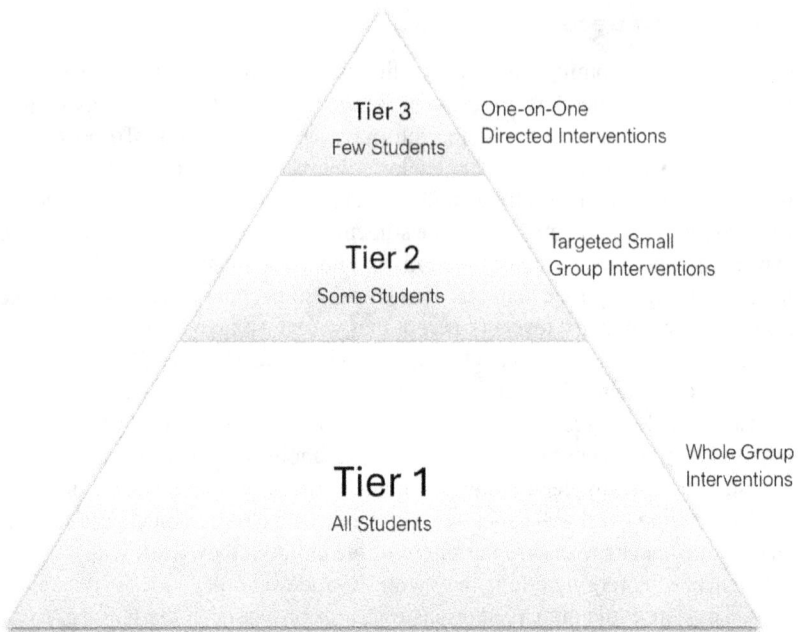

Figure 9.1 Students' social–emotional competencies can be supported by educators at all three tiers.

There are many programs that schools can implement to promote social–emotional competencies in students. Such programs are collectively called social-emotional learning or SEL programs. Common SEL programs include Leader in Me, Second Step, and Zones of Regulation (Bergin et al., 2024). Such programs – in preschool through high schools – can increase social–emotional competence and raise grades and test scores (Cipriano et al., 2023).

SEL programs are generally designed to be implemented by teachers with all the students in their classroom. However, some programs may be designed for targeted students who have specific skill gaps. Educators often use a pyramid model called a *multi-tiered system of support* (Sailor et al., 2020) to describe different levels of support for different students. It can be applied to academics (e.g., reading instruction) or to social–emotional well-being and behavior. See Figure 9.1.

- Tier 1, at the base of the pyramid, is universal, schoolwide support provided to all students and typically delivered by the classroom teacher. A majority (about 80%–90%) of students respond well to this support.

- Tier 2 involves additional structured supports using specialized interventions for targeted students, often delivered or overseen by school counselors, social workers, special education teachers, or other specialists. Tier 2 generally meets the needs of identified students (about 5%–15%) who do not respond effectively to Tier 1 supports.
- Tier 3 involves intensive, individualized interventions, often delivered by a team of specialists that includes a psychologist (see Chapter 11). Tier 3 is designed to meet the needs of identified students (about 1%–5%) who do not respond effectively to Tier 1 or 2 supports.

Tier 1 research-based strategies that are implemented effectively in general classrooms can help students who need Tier 2 or 3 supports by creating a safe, warm, inclusive environment. Although they focus on promoting social–emotional competencies in all students, Tier 1 strategies may be most beneficial for high-risk students. Tier 1 supports do not replace Tier 2 or 3 interventions, but they may minimize mental health needs and increase the success of Tier 2 and 3 interventions. Educators need to be trained, supported, and certified to deliver interventions at all three tiers. Research finds that qualified professionals are significantly more effective than untrained persons at promoting students' well-being.

Promoting Emotional Competence

When you help students with their own self-regulation of emotion, you also help them read others' emotions. This is because students need to be able to contain their own emotions in order to accurately perceive others' emotions and anticipate how their behavior can affect others' emotions. Let's discuss how to promote each aspect of emotional competence next.

Regulating One's Own Emotions

Regardless of one's role or field, anyone who works with infants through emerging adults can use the general strategies that we discuss at the end of Chapters 3–6 to help students regulate their own emotions. Those that apply to educators include:

1. Use inductive discipline. Students become angry when power assertion is used.
2. Talk about emotions. Help students learn to label their emotions. You can do this when opportunities naturally occur. For example, you might say "Derek's feels hurt because you didn't include him in your group. How would you feel if you were him?" Or, you can talk about emotions when discussing participants in historical events or characters in novels. Especially, focus on

discussing and expressing gratitude because feelings of gratitude improve mood and lead to being more prosocial toward others (not just the person we feel gratitude toward). Talk about how much you value kindness and helping. Point out the prosocial behavior of characters in books, media, and real-life.

3. Create an emotionally upbeat environment where mostly positive emotions are experienced, but where it is also safe to express authentic, reasonable negative emotions such as occasional frustration or anger. Positive teacher–student and student–student relationships are key to an upbeat classroom.
4. Respond appropriately to students. Validate their feelings (but not necessarily their behavior if it is harmful or disruptive.) Help students use constructive coping strategies (see Box 1.1). Don't forget that reappraisal is often (but not always) the best coping strategy for situations that students cannot control.
5. Co-regulate students who have not yet learned to control their emotions. Help them soothe big emotions. Educators who work with young children should refer to Chapter 3 for specific strategies with preschoolers.
6. Teach good sleep habits. Sleep deprivation is a key cause of emotional problems.

There are programs designed to teach emotion regulation in schools. For example, in the R.U.L.E.R. (Recognizing, Understanding, Labeling, Expressing, and Regulating emotions) program, a key task is to learn to label feelings accurately. It uses the "Mood Meter" to help students plot emotions on a grid of energy and pleasantness. Students and teachers create a document that outlines how they want to feel in their classroom. The "Meta-Moment" helps students stop and think about constructive coping strategies before reacting impulsively. Students learn conflict resolution. Teachers are trained to use the program. Another example of a program is the PATHS curriculum discussed in Chapter 8. It is used in schools to teach students emotion self-regulation and to read others' emotions.

Students who have significant problems regulating their own emotions may have an emotional disorder, such as anxiety or depression (see Chapter 1). Educators should advocate for psychological help for such students (see Chapters 10 and 11).

Reading Others' Emotions

Students at all ages will use social referencing and emotion contagion to read others' emotions. This means they will catch an educator's enthusiasm (or boredom) for a topic. For example, a teacher greeted 12-year-olds entering his class with a big smile and a twinkle in his eye. He said, "We have a really cool experiment to do today!" Most students immediately broke into a smile and asked, "What is it!?" mirroring his enthusiasm. Students are more likely to adopt the emotions of teachers they like.

You can help students read others' emotions better, and build their theory of mind skills, when you converse with them about others' feelings and mental states. You can do this when natural opportunities arise, such as Derek's hurt feelings, or during lessons. For example, while reading Anne Frank's *The Diary of a Young Girl,* you might discuss what Anne Frank *felt, thought, believed, hoped, guessed, expected* while hiding in an attic for 2 years. Such discussion can help build students' ability to understand others' minds and hearts. Also, recall that a powerful way to promote empathy and compassion toward others is to use other-oriented inductive discipline, including pointing out to students how their behavior made others' feel.

Promoting Social Competence

The more students feel peer support and teacher support in the school, the more motivated students, especially teens, are to learn. Let's discuss this next.

Increase Friendship

Friendship in schools is important. Compared to students who have no friends, students who have a friend in a classroom feel more like they belong, and they behave more prosocially and less aggressively toward classmates. Teachers can promote friendships by seating friendless students near prosocial leaders and by pointing out positive attributes of the student to others. Positive attributes could include artistic ability, knowledge about a specific topic (like dinosaurs or musicians,) academic competence, or athletic ability. If a teacher praises a student, the student's popularity will increase over time; if a teacher disciplines or criticizes a student, the student may become more rejected.

There are also programs that target specific students (Tier 2) to build friendship skills. One such program is "Fast Friends" (Echols & Ivanich, 2021). Students are brought together in three sessions. In the first two sessions, they ask each other 36 questions that progress from impersonal ("What's your favorite food") to more personal ("What's something you will do differently from your parents?"). In the third session, they solve a puzzle together. The program helps students, across ethnic/racial groups, develop friendships. Recall that the best predictor of being liked by peers and having high-quality friendships is prosocial behavior. Let's look at how educators can affect prosocial behavior next.

Increase Prosocial Behavior

Helping students increase their prosocial is important because they learn more in schools that have a prosocial culture, particularly low-income students

(Berkowitz et al., 2017). Three powerhouse strategies that teachers can use to increase prosocial behavior in students are the following: (1) Use inductive discipline when students misbehave, particularly other-oriented induction. Review Chapter 4 for how to do this. (2) Praise students when they behave prosocially toward each other. (3) Build teacher-student relationships (TSRs). A program called ProsocialEd trains teachers to do this (Bergin, 2018). As a result of using the ProsocialEd program, teachers enjoy teaching more, students become more prosocial, and teachers and students develop better relationships. Let's talk about praise next, and then we'll discuss TSRs.

Praise Prosocial Behavior

Imagine you are a sixth grade teacher and a student, Issac, just had his backpack zipper pull apart so that everything fell out of the pack. Some students rush to help pick up all his spilled belongings. You say, "Raul, Derek, and Sonja, you are so kind for helping Issac. Good job!" It is important to publicly praise students in this way so that other students notice the prosocial behavior. This communicates that you value and notice prosocial behavior, setting a standard for the classroom. This also communicates that Raul, Derek, and Sonja are kind people, which will make classmates like them better and make them feel better about themselves, motivating them to be more prosocial in the future.

Research has found that when teachers increase the amount of praise they give students, relative to the number of reprimands, the students become more cooperative, less disruptive, and earn higher grades. This works even for highly disruptive students (Caldarella et al., 2020). Most teachers give one statement of praise for every four to nine reprimands or negative statements. If teachers can change that balance to one praise for one reprimand, student behavior improves dramatically.

Some educators want to give students rewards (e.g., stickers, candy, points) for prosocial behavior. Yet, this actually *undermines* prosocial behavior over the long-term. Why? It feels overly controlling to students, decreases their motivation to be prosocial, and undermines their development of self-control. In a famous experiment, preschoolers who liked to draw were randomly assigned to a group that was rewarded for their drawing or to a control group that was not rewarded. Later, the children who received the reward showed *less* interest in drawing. This effect has been replicated many times with children, teens, and adults doing many different tasks (e.g., Murayama, 2022). In contrast, praise does not have this undermining effect, so use praise but not rewards to acknowledge students' prosocial behaviors.

Build Positive Teacher–Student Relationships (TSRs)

Research robustly shows the importance of positive TSRs. If students have a positive relationship with their teachers, they are more engaged in class and learn more. Students are motivated to work hard for teachers who care for them. Students are also less aggressive and more prosocial in classrooms where they have positive TSRs. Students who experience positive TSRs are less likely to be retained, referred for special education, truant, suspended, or drop-out (Olivier & Archambault, 2017). Furthermore, when a teacher is supportive of a student, even if the student is rejected by classmates, the student is likely to become less anxious and depressed (Spilt et al., 2014). And the student isn't likely to be rejected for long because classmates come to like students better who have positive TSRs. All students benefit from positive TSRs, but they are especially important for low-income or racially minoritized students, at-risk boys, and for children who have insecure attachment to their own parents. See Box 9.1.

Box 9.1   Interview of an Educator

Riley is a veteran educator who currently works as a coach and mentor to novice school administrators. She says all educators need to know about social–emotional development so that they can work effectively with the whole child and not just teach them academics. She also believes educators can make a difference in students' social–emotional competencies. Riley tells novice administrators that relationship strategies are their best tools.

Research supports several strategies that will help you improve relationships with students. Two strategies that we've already discussed – praising students for being prosocial and using inductive discipline, rather than power assertion (see Chapter 4) – both lead to more positive relationships with students. We all like people better who affirm us and treat us with respect. In addition, you should be sensitive and responsive toward students. Frequently have positive, warm interactions. Make sure students feel seen and heard. Reading this book will help because adults who know more about child development tend to be more sensitive toward children. Find something you share with specific students, such as a favorite sports team, hobby, or interest (e.g., reading fantasy books, bike riding, specific musicians).

In addition to these general strategies that work with most children, there are specific interventions that can help you build positive TSRs with challenging students. First, get another teacher to be a reflective partner. Tell the other teacher what behaviors irritate you about the student. Then, describe the exact same behaviors from the student's perspective. This helps you develop empathy and energizes you to generate possible solutions (Gehlbach et al., 2023). Second, use the 2×10 strategy where you spen 2 minutes for 10 days getting to know the challenging student better (McKibben, 2014). Third, tell the student what you admire about them by using specific anecdotes.

Some children are easier to develop positive relationships with; for example, children who have *secure attachment to their parents* are easier. They tend to have higher academic achievement, more willingness to take on challenging tasks, and greater ability to get along well with others. In contrast, insecure students tend to be aggressive, anxious, or disruptive. They have learned from their parents that adults cannot be trusted to consistently care for them or that adults are hostile and rejecting. However, if educators can manage to disconfirm the students' beliefs by being responsive, warm, and supportive, the students are likely to become less aggressive, anxious, or disruptive over time. This doesn't happen overnight; it typically takes at least several months. Positive TSRs also help *teachers* enjoy teaching more, and they teach better because they are motivated by positive relationships with their students.

Reduce Antisocial Behavior

When teachers use the strategies described above to promote students' prosocial behavior, they also reduce aggression. This is important because aggressive students do not fare well in school; they have attention and learning problems and earn lower grades and test scores. This occurs as early as kindergarten but is especially true in high school. If the strategies described above are not sufficient, specialist educators may be called upon to help aggressive students. Usually, these educators have special training and may be counselors, school psychologists, or special education teachers. They may use an intervention called *behavior modification*, which is based on principles of behaviorism (see Chapter 7). Behavior modification involves taking the following steps:

1. Collect data on the problem behaviors. When do they occur? What happens before the behaviors, and what consequences follow that might be reinforcing the behavior? For example, a child gets out of math class for misbehavior because they are sent to the safe room where they do not have to do math. This is reinforcing to the child who doesn't like math and will usually increase misbehavior.
2. Systematically alter the situation and see what happens. Can you change what is causing the behavior?
3. Set goals with the child for improved behavior.
4. Reinforce positive behavior. Give the child praise or feedback for improvement.

You might be wondering where the punishment is in this sequence. Most educators try to avoid punishment because it can cause resentment and aggression, it doesn't teach replacement behaviors, and it provides a bad model for students to imitate. It is power assertive (see Chapter 4). Instead, if correction is needed, use inductive discipline.

Some programs are designed for students with behavioral challenges. These are called "behavioral" programs to distinguish them from SEL programs. Common interventions are PBIS (Positive Behavior Intervention Support) and BIST (Behavior Intervention Support Team). BIST begins with the principle that students with behavior challenges have not yet learned to behave appropriately in school. Students who need help are identified, taught clear expectations for behavior, and given feedback and practice for those behaviors. BIST strongly emphasizes building trusting relationships between adults and students. Students are held accountable for misbehavior, but adults communicate that they are there to help the student learn self-control.

Promoting a Healthy Sense of Self

Varied personalities in a classroom are part of what makes being an educator so enjoyable. However, some personality attributes (Chapter 4) are a better fit to school settings than others. The personality attribute *conscientiousness* is an asset in school settings; it consistently predicts higher grades and test scores starting as early as age 3 and into emerging adulthood (Mammadov, 2022). On the other hand, the personality attribute *high activity level* can be a challenge in schools that expect students to sit still for long periods. Other personality traits (e.g., *extraversion* and *shyness*) do not affect how well children do in school. The role of educators is to make the classroom or school environment as good a fit as possible for children's varied personalities. For example, it is useful to give children with high activity levels movement breaks.

Build Healthy Self-Esteem

Students with high self-esteem tend to earn higher grades and test scores, which in turn increase self-esteem. So, what can educators do to promote high self-esteem in students? Some of the same things we've already discussed: (1) Build positive TSRs. (2) Use inductive discipline. (3) Increase prosocial and decrease antisocial behavior. (4) Praise students when you catch them being good. In addition, when you help students become more competent – whether in academics, sports, or social settings – you promote their self-esteem. Be careful not to tell children that they are more competent than they are because this leads to mistrust. Instead, point out their improvement and scaffold them on how to improve even more, as Eduardo the swim coach did in Chapter 6. Recall that he tells students, "I saw how you improved your breathing technique. That's great! But your stroke needs work. Focus on stretching your arm like this." Eduardo is a beloved coach; all his swimmers think they are his favorite!

Promote Healthy Ethnic Identity

Part of healthy self-identity is to feel good about your ethnic/racial group. Minoritized students who have a positive ethnic identity tend to have higher grades and test scores, like and feel bonded to school, and complete more education (Butler-Barns et al., 2016). Research suggests that educators can promote positive ethnic identities in five ways: (1) Do not tolerate gender or racial harassment. (2) Treat all students fairly. (3) Hold high expectations and give supportive feedback that communicates "I have high expectations for you, and I know that you can reach them." (4) Promote contact between groups and cross-race friendships where students pursue cooperative goals together. (5) Talk about the contributions and value of different groups.

Chapter Summary

Education takes place in many settings such as vocational training institutions, community colleges, universities, sports teams, and medical training. Educators, that is, people who provide education to others, are key promoters of social–emotional development. Unfortunately, there is a great need for promotion of social–emotional development because K-12 students have increased in disruptive behavior and mental health challenges for about 50 years; the trend started well before the COVID-19 pandemic. Multi-tiered systems of support can promote students' social–emotional competencies. Educators who work with infants through emerging adults can use the general strategies that are discussed in Chapters 3–6, and implement special SEL or behavioral programs. The more peers and teachers support each other socially and emotionally, the more motivated students are to learn.

References

Bergin, C. (2018). *Designing a prosocial classroom: Fostering collaboration in students from pre-K-12 with the curriculum you already use*. Norton.

Bergin, C., Tsai, C., Prewett, S., Jones, E., Bergin, D., & Murphy, B. (2024). Effectiveness of a social-emotional learning program for both teachers and students. *AERA Open, 10*(1), 1–18.

Berkowitz, R., Moore, H., Astor, R. A., & Benbenishty, R. (2017). A research synthesis of the associations between socioeconomic background, inequality, school climate, and academic achievement. *Review of Educational Research, 87*(2), 425–469.

Butler-Barnes, S. T., Varner, F., Williams, A., & Sellers, R. (2016). Academic identity: A longitudinal investigation of African American adolescents' academic persistence. *Journal of Black Psychology, 43*(7), 714–739.

Caldarella, P., Larsen, R. A. A., Williams, L., Downs, K. R., Wills, H. P., & Wehby, J. H. (2020). Effects of teachers' praise-to-reprimand ratios on elementary students' on-task behaviour. *Educational Psychology, 40*(10), 1306–1322.

Cipriano, C., Strambler, M. J., Naples, L. H., Ha, C., Kirk, M., Wood, M., Sehgal, K., Zieher, A. K., Eveleigh, A., McCarthy, M., Funaro, M., Ponnock, A., Chow, J. C., & Durlak, J. (2023). The state of evidence for social and emotional learning: A contemporary meta-analysis of universal school-based SEL interventions. *Child Development, 94*(5), 1181–1204.

Echols, L. & Ivanich, J. (2021). From "Fast Friends" to true friends: Can a contact intervention promote friendships in middle school? *Journal of Research on Adolescence, 31*(4), 1152–1171.

Gehlbach, H., Mascio, B., & McIntyre, J. (2023). Social perspective taking: A professional development induction to improve teacher–student relationships and student learning. *Journal of Educational Psychology, 115*(2), 330–348.

Irwin, V., Wang, K., Cui, J., & Thompson, A. (2022). *Report on indicators of school crime and safety: 2021* (NCES 2022-092/NCJ 304625). U.S. Department of Education.

Mammadov, S. (2022). Big Five personality traits and academic performance: A meta-analysis. *Journal of Personality, 90*(2), 222–255.

McKibben, S. (2014, July 1). *The two-minute relationship builder*. ASCD. www.ascd.org/el/articles/the-two-minute-relationship-builder

Murayama, K. (2022). A reward-learning framework of knowledge acquisition: An integrated account of curiosity, interest, and intrinsic–extrinsic rewards. *Psychological Review, 129*(1), 175–198.

Olivier, E., & Archambault, I. (2017). Hyperactivity, inattention, and student engagement: The protective role of relationships with teachers and peers. *Learning and Individual Differences, 59*, 86–95.

Sailor, W., Skrtic, T. M., Cohn, M., & Olmstead, C. (2020). Preparing teacher educators for statewide scale-up of Multi-Tiered System of Support (MTSS). *Teacher Education and Special Education, 44*(1), 24–41.

Spilt, J. L., van Lier, P. A. C., Leflot, G., Onghena, P., & Colpin, H. (2014). Children's social self-concept and internalizing problems: The influence of peers and teachers. *Child Development, 85*(3), 1248–1256.

Chapter 10

Promoting Social and Emotional Competence in Social Work

Leslie is a social worker. Remember from Box 1.3 that she worked in an after-school setting with youth who needed to learn social–emotional competencies. She worked as part of a team. After working in this setting for a few years, she earned a license to become an LCSW (Licensed Clinical Social Worker). This allowed her to open a private practice to provide therapy with patients on a one-to-one basis, or for families. She works primarily through telehealth, meaning her meetings with clients are virtual. Her clients are primarily adolescents to emerging adults.

In this chapter, we will discuss how social–emotional skills and concepts affect social work settings. Social work is an emotionally rewarding and emotionally taxing career field (Engstrom, 2019). The work can be very demanding, often with large workloads and complex duties. However, the nature of social work provides opportunities to deeply serve others.

Who Is a Social Worker?

Social workers work in many fields such as health, education, psychology, psychiatry, child protection, adoption, child welfare, foster care, law/justice, shelters for battered women, and others. They may work in teams or alone (Axelrad-Levy et al., 2023). Duties may include relationship building, referring to outside resources, assisting children and families with transitions, placing children in agencies or families, ensuring the safety of children, counseling children and families, helping families adjust to crises or health diagnoses, and other related duties. Social workers may focus primarily on case management or provide therapy. In addition to Leslie in the opening vignette, some examples of social workers include the following:

1. Kendra works in a school to help children with difficult home situations. She works with the guardians of the children to create a supportive home environment so that the children can be successful at school and with peers.

DOI: 10.4324/9781003046455-10

2. Alejandro works in a hospital to help families of youth with chronic illnesses understand the treatment plan and get the community resources (e.g., support groups and homecare services) they need to manage the illness.
3. Travis works with youth who have been arrested or are on probation to develop rehabilitation plans and connect them to community resources to prevent further arrests.

Social workers may work with children and families in governmental and non-profit agencies. They often intervene when there is a disruption in the family unit, such as being an advocate for children in divorce cases. Teleworking, that is, providing care using electronic media like video calls instead of in-person visits, is increasingly common and increased because of the COVID-19 pandemic. While telework can be convenient for many workers, it also carries the risk of burnout due to emotional disconnection from fellow workers and from clients (Kranke et al., 2024).

How Do You Become a Social Worker?

Social workers typically have a bachelor's or master's degree, and a few have a doctorate. The level of education required depends on the role of the social worker. Social workers with bachelor's degrees may work in adoption, child welfare, foster care, education, child protection, and related fields. This kind of work is typically done in teams with a supervisor. You may be assigned a caseload of children or families with whom you work.

Licensed clinical social workers must have a master's or doctoral degree, complete supervised clinical work, and pass a licensure exam. Clinical social workers are more likely to work in health or law and related fields than general social workers (Biddle et al., 2018). Some clinical social workers may have supervisors who are doctoral-level psychologists or medical physicians, or they may have a private practice, such as Leslie in the opening vignette.

How Do Social Workers Promote Social–Emotional Competence in Children and Youth?

Social workers often work with children and families, so it is important for them to understand how children's social–emotional competencies develop and how to promote those competencies. Social workers may train and coach other adults to foster social–emotional competencies in children under their care, such as coaching parents or supporting teachers. In addition, social workers must have strong social–emotional skills themselves because they need to build trusting, supportive relationships with clients so that clients feel safe to work through challenges.

Social workers typically collaborate with others, such as healthcare providers, teachers, and psychologists, to address the multiple needs of clients, often being the coordinator of care among the varied providers. They are advocates for their clients' rights and needs in the community. They may focus primarily on case management and/or providing therapy.

Recall from Chapter 9 that educators apply different levels of support to students depending on their level of need. Tier 1 is schoolwide instruction provided to all students and typically delivered by the classroom teacher, Tier 2 is a little more targeted and is applied to students who do not respond effectively to Tier 1, and Tier 3 involves intensive, individualized intervention that is often delivered by a team of specialists. Social workers can work with children at any of the three tiers of intervention (Chapter 9) but are most likely to work with children needing Tier 2 or 3 intervention. Examples of Tier 1 interventions that involve social workers include improving high-school students' attitudes toward sexually inappropriate behavior, sexual assault, and sexual harassment; postponing onset of sexual intercourse for middle- and high-school students; reducing aggression in elementary-school students; and improving stress management in sixth graders. Examples of Tier 2 interventions for targeted at-risk students include cognitive behavioral therapy (CBT) to improve self-control and classroom behavior, improving emotional awareness and coping skills, and addressing attitude change regarding body image and self-esteem (Allen-Meares et al., 2013).

Social workers must be culturally competent and sensitive to their clients' diverse backgrounds. Let's see what Akiva, a social worker, does to support a refugee family of nine – with two parents, six children, and one grandmother. The family is dealing with language barriers, cultural differences, and trauma from escaping a war zone. Akiva first met with the family and thoroughly assessed current needs. She then provided several services:

1. Teaching cultural education to help the family navigate their new community and cultural norms.
2. Finding permanent housing and a job for the father that resulted in work at a grocery store.
3. Connecting to a church group that provided home goods for refugees to get beds and clothing.
4. Connecting to English language learner services for the school-age children.
5. Providing trauma-informed therapy that included play therapy for the children.

This kind of wholistic care that *addresses multiple needs* of the family is common in social work and likely to result in an improvement in the children's social–emotional well-being over time despite their trauma. See Box 10.1.

Promoting Emotional Competence

Unfortunately, many children experience trauma, like Akiva's refugee family, or live in neglectful, harsh, or abusive families. In these circumstances, children may not learn emotion regulation skills or may learn destructive emotion patterns. They need therapists' help to learn more adaptive coping strategies. Social workers may use the same general strategies that we discussed at the end of Chapters 3–6. That is, they may help clients develop healthy emotion regulation by talking about emotions so that clients learn to label and understand their emotions. They may help clients use constructive coping strategies (Box 1.1) to deal with overwhelming emotions. The reappraisal coping strategy is particularly helpful when clients cannot control the situation. They may teach optimistic thinking when appropriate. They may also help clients address underlying causes of emotional problems.

Much of what therapists do is "talk" therapy in which therapist and client talk about problems and how to overcome them. However, young children need a different kind of therapy because their language and planning skills are still developing. In addition, while attachment is healthy for children, it can make it a challenge for social workers to work with young children who are wary of non-attachement figures (AFs). What can you do to get a wary toddler to cooperate with you? Give them time to warm up to you. Offer them something, then take it when they offer it back. Play peek-a-boo. Such "give-and-take" games make them more willing to cooperate with you. Be sure to give them control over the approach and follow their lead. If a toddler backs away, you back away until they invite you closer. Also, ask the parent to smile at you. Children use social referencing (Chapter 1) to see whether the parent believes you are safe. Leave the child in physical contact with the preferred AF while you play warm-up games.

You can also use play therapy with young children (see Figure 10.1). Play allows children to express themselves, explore feelings, and make sense of their experiences. In play therapy, the child leads the play while the social worker observes and interacts as needed. A wide range of toys and supplies (e.g., building blocks, dress-up clothes, art supplies, dolls) are available. Children express their emotions and work through traumatic experiences through play. Play therapy has been shown to reduce anxiety, depression, and aggression. It can also help children work through guilt. You might wonder why a young child would feel guilt, but toddlers are not always good at judging whether they "caused" an event. This can lead them to feel guilty about things that are not their fault, such as when their parents fight. As a result, young children are vulnerable to misplaced guilt.

In Chapter 3, you learned about typical patterns of tantrums in young children. Tantrums that are out of this normal developmental pattern can be a red flag for emotional disorders. What should you watch for? Watch for extreme or

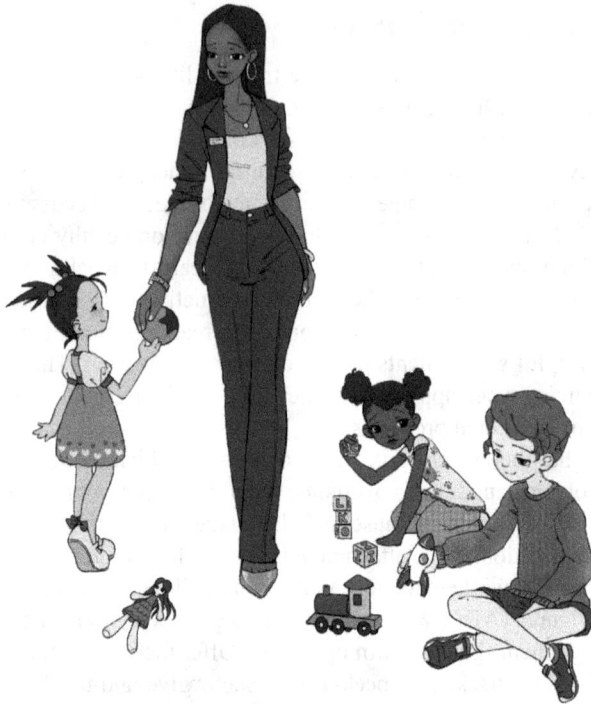

Figure 10.1 Play therapy is useful with young children to help them express thoughts and feelings.

frequent tantrums that are long (e.g., over 15 minutes), involve hurting other people, are "out of the blue," are aimed at non-parental adults, and are followed by intense shame or guilt. These patterns of tantrums warrant attention and possible therapeutic help from a social worker or psychologist. Beyond the toddler years, frequent tantrums in preschoolers also warrant attention. However, do not worry if there is a brief spike in tantrums when a major stressor occurs, such as a family move, as long as it is temporary.

Box 10.1   Interview with a Social Worker

Timothy is a social worker. He says that knowledge, understanding, and application are the cornerstones of good social work practice. He suggests that new social workers read many sources and then translate what they have read into practical tools and techniques to help their clients.

They should also confer with colleagues, even after they have many years of experience. He also advises social workers to learn about and understand all environments that their clients inhabit. "Don't be afraid to see the world the way your client does." Timothy learned about social–emotional competence during 5.5 years of graduate study in clinical psychology and social work. He says that "learning about social–emotional competence is critical for all social workers. I truly believe this. It is crucial for working with clients, especially children."

Promoting Social Competence

In Chapter 3, you learned that attachment affects many important outcomes. If you work consistently over time with the same children, you can establish an attachment-like relationship. However, it is not easy to do with children who have learned from their parents that others cannot be trusted to consistently care for them. Because insecure attachment is foundational to social–emotional disorders, social workers need to counter the clients' experience that adults are insensitive and unresponsive. Changing children's internal working models can take several months or longer. To promote a secure relationship with the children with whom you work, you need to be consistent and responsive, rather than detached or critical with children. They need to have warm, positive interactions. Their parents should also read this book! Adults with greater knowledge of children's development tend to be more sensitive toward them. Social workers may train parents to help them create more nurturing environments, promote secure attachment, or use more effective discipline.

Peer Support

Social workers develop intervention plans that use different kinds of techniques to build social–emotional skills in clients. This may include counseling with clients, referring clients to other services, and doing skill-building activities. One approach they may use in a variety of settings, such as shelters, schools, or hospitals, is peer-support groups. For example, they might provide social skills training to a group of peers, such as how to initiate a conversation or resolve conflicts. The group can role play with each other. Social workers may help children with Autism Spectrum Disorder learn skills to navigate social interactions with peers. Social workers may implement anti-bullying or peer mentoring programs in schools.

Peer-support programs are often used with emerging adults. Peers who have experienced and overcome a challenge can encourage those who are experiencing similar challenges. For example, programs may focus on substance misuse treatment or may focus on helping emerging adults transition to independence. The peers build supportive relationships as they help each other acquire the skills needed for adult roles (e.g., independent living, employment, relationships). Such peer-support groups give individuals hope, build relationships, and help clients feel less loneliness or shame. Peer-support programs are typically part of a wholistic array of services provided by a team that may be coordinated by a social worker.

Friendship Skills

Therapy for children and youth may center on helping very shy, aggressive, or otherwise socially unskilled children develop the skills they need to make and keep friends. In Chapter 4, you learned how important friendships are for children's happiness, coping with stress, and engagement in school. One strategy social workers use is to help children see things from another's perspective – that is reading others' emotions and developing theory of mind skills. This involves the therapist asking the same kinds of questions that you ask when using other-oriented inductive discipline (see Chapter 4): "How do you think he felt when you did that?" Or, "Why do you think she did that?" Another strategy is talking about emotions. "She seemed very angry." Or, "Do you think it made him sad when you did that?" A third strategy is to help children reappraise the situation when a friend has made them angry. Rather than assume the friend is deliberately being mean, you can say "Perhaps she misunderstood" or "Maybe he was just trying to do something else."

A fourth strategy is to directly coach friendship-making skills. One example is to coach clients and their parents on how to invite a friend over to play; then be ready with a list of two to four things they would like to do with their friend. That way, when the awkward "What do you want to do?" "I don't know, what do you want to do" conversation occurs, the child can move past it. Another example is to coach a child in how to enter an ongoing group. This is a difficult social skill; even adults can find this daunting. Just bursting into the group disrupts the group and could lead to rejection. A better approach is to take it gradually. First hover, listen to what the topic is. Then, contribute a brief affirming comment or ask a question on the topic. Then, fully join the group. Very shy children might be taught how to look at someone and say "Hi [name]." If youth are in destructive friendships, the social worker might guide the child through questioning: "Does she bring out your best self?" "How do you feel when you are with him?" "Do you feel comfortable being yourself with her?" Then, the social worker may walk the client through identifying more positive others who share the client's interests and with whom they may become friends.

Promoting Self-Esteem

Recall that one of the components of self-esteem is having valued skills. Some occupational social workers help emerging adult clients develop skills that make them feel more capable. They coach clients through setting realistic goals. (Unattainable goals are likely to make clients feel like failures.) They help clients distinguish between *their* goals and *expectations put on them* by family and friends. They may help clients learn how to get training, where to get it, and how to afford it. They may help clients with disabilities navigate community resources to build self-sufficiency.

Chapter Summary

Social work is an emotionally rewarding and emotionally taxing career field that provides opportunities to deeply serve individuals and communities. Social workers work in a variety of fields. They may work in teams or alone. Social workers may focus primarily on case management and/or providing therapy. In schools, social workers may be involved with Tier 1, 2, or 3 interventions. They work with children, youth, and adults from widely varied backgrounds, so they must be culturally competent. They provide wholistic care that addresses multiple needs of individuals and families. To help clients develop social–emotional competencies, social workers use a variety of approaches including play therapy with young children or peer support groups with emerging adults.

References

Allen-Meares, P., Montgomery, K., & Kim, J. (2013). School-based social work interventions: A cross-national systematic review. *Social Work, 58*(3), 253–262.

Axelrad-Levy, T., Schwartz Tayri, T.M., Achdut, N., & Sarid, O. (2023). The perceived job performance of child welfare workers during the COVID-19 pandemic. *Clinical Social Work Journal, 51*(2), 175–187.

Biddle, K., Harven, A., & Hudley, C. (2018). *Careers in child and adolescent development: a student's guide to working in the field.* Routledge.

Engstrom, S. (2019). Interpersonal justice: The importance of relationships for child and family social workers. *Journal of Social Work Practice, 33*(1), 41–53

Kranke, D. A., Barmaksezian, N., Milligan, S., & Der-Martirosian, C. (2024). Countering burnout associated with teleworking in this postpandemic era. *Social Work, 69*(2), 197–200.

Chapter 11

Applying Social and Emotional Competence in Psychology

Who Is a Psychologist?

There are two very broad categories of psychologists who deal with the development of social–emotional competence in children and adults: *research* and *applied* psychologists. Applied psychologists work directly with clients who need extra support to develop social–emotional competence. They may work in schools, hospitals, or private offices.

Research psychologists conduct research. One group, *developmental psychologists*, studies age trends in children, such as what changes in social–emotional competence at different ages. For example, how does emotion regulation change from age 2 to 22? They also study individual and group differences in social–emotional competence, including what are the causes and the results of those differences among children. For example, how are boys and girls different in emotion regulation? Or, how is Tom different from Jose in emotion regulation, why are they different, and how might that difference affect their long-term well-being? There are thousands of developmental psychologists across the world who conduct this research, including the authors of this book. Some other types of research psychologists might specialize in studying specific areas of development. For example,

- *Cognitive* psychologists study mental processes like problem-solving, memory, creativity.
- *Educational* psychologists study learning, in or out of formal school settings.
- *Health* psychologists study the intersection of psychological and physical health.
- *Sport* psychologists study the psychology of sports and how to help athletes perform well.
- *Neuropsychologists* study the intersection of behavior and the brain.

We've drawn a line between research and applied psychologists to make the distinction clear. However, the distinction can be a little fuzzy. For example, some

DOI: 10.4324/9781003046455-11

developmental psychologists (like the authors) use research to develop and test applied interventions that improve social–emotional competencies in youth. For another example, some clinical psychologists conduct research on what types of therapy work best. Thus, you can be both a research and applied psychologist, although many specialize in only conducting research or only providing an application like therapy.

This book presents a summary of the research of developmental psychologists, although it is a brief summary. For example, there are many thousands of studies on just the topic of attachment. Nevertheless, because previous sections of this book focus on the work of research psychologists, the remainder of this chapter will focus on the work of applied psychologists.

How Do You Become a Psychologist?

To become a research psychologist, you must earn a doctorate (PhD) and work in either a university or research institute (sometimes called a "think tank"). It takes 7–11 years of university education to learn to be a research psychologist because you must not only master existing research content but also learn the skills to conduct new research. We find it deeply interesting work!

To become an applied psychologist, you have to earn either a master's degree or doctorate, depending on which specialty you choose. For example,

- Counselors typically work in schools, focusing on career counseling or helping youth cope with life challenges. A master's degree is required.
- Licensed Clinical Social Workers (LCSW) treat clients with mental health disorders, trauma, relationship challenges, or substance abuse. A master's degree plus supervised field work are required.
- School psychologists work in schools to help children with academic and social–emotional issues. A doctorate is required.
- Pediatric psychologists help children deal with medical treatment or health issues, often working in a hospital setting. A doctorate is required.
- Clinical psychologists treat patients with serious behavior and mental health challenges. A doctorate is required.

How Do Psychologists Promote Social–Emotional Competence in Children and Youth?

Psychologists can work with children at any of the three tiers of intervention (see Chapter 9) but are most likely to work with children needing Tier 3 intervention. Some clients at this level are prescribed medications for their condition, but because medication can have serious side effects, most experts recommend psychotherapy first for youth. Psychologists help clients with both social and emotional challenges.

Promoting Emotional Competence

Emotionally competent children are predominantly positive. Children who are chronically sad, angry, or moody may need intervention. Poor emotion regulation is a foundation of mental health challenges. In fact, "irritability" – which means becoming angry and frustrated too easily – is a common reason for children being referred for psychological services. But also remember that by age 10, most children can hide or "fake" emotions. Children can be distressed by something (e.g., being bullied at school or having parents' divorce) but pretend they are not, so it is important to be alert to emotional disorders. Generally, the sooner emotional disorders are treated, the more successful the treatment.

Psychologists may work with children who experience abuse. The abuse can lead to either tightly over-regulated emotions or under-regulated intense anger, fear, and shame. It may lead to depression. It may also lead to hypersensitivity to reading anger in others, which helps keep children safe from abusers but makes it difficult to read other's emotions accurately. Therapy can help abused youth learn strategies for coping with anger, grief, and shame associated with abuse.

Psychologists may also work with children who have anxiety and depression. These are common emotional disorders and are becoming more common. Rates of anxiety and depression have been rising for decades (e.g., Krokstad et al., 2022; Parodi et al., 2022), with a worldwide spike during the COVID-19 pandemic (Santomauro et al., 2021). A child with *anxiety* is worried about future threats or threats to the sense of self. A child with *depression* feels sadness that is severe for at least 2 weeks or that is mild but long-term. Children with anxiety and depression have trouble upregulating positive emotions and downregulating negative emotions and may not be able to flexibly use different coping strategies (Gross & Jazaieri, 2014). Anxiety and depression may have some of the same symptoms, such as poor concentration or fidgety behavior, but also some differences. For example, feeling worthless, being self-critical, and crying frequently are more typical of depression than anxiety. Half of children who will have these internalizing disorders are diagnosed by age 6 (for anxiety) or 11 (for depression). One caution is that young children can seem anxious and wary but not have an anxiety disorder. About a third of seemingly anxious preschoolers will outgrow it in middle childhood. Depression, in contrast, becomes *more* prevalent in mid-adolescence, but then decreases. Anyone can be anxious or depressed at times, but those with emotional disorders have chronic, intense symptoms that interfere with daily functioning. Anxiety and depression are linked to other disorders, such as ADHD, learning disorders, eating disorders, loneliness, friendlessness, and low grades or test scores.

A primary cause of both anxiety and depression (as well as *externalizing* disorders) is insecure attachment (Deneault et al., 2021). Research robustly finds that insecure attachment predicts these emotional disorders from infancy to adulthood. Perhaps this is because if children do not believe their parents will be there to meet their needs, they will feel chronic anxiety. In addition, if children's parents are insensitive to them, they will not learn to regulate their emotions. Other aspects of parenting also predict poor emotion regulation, such as parents being negative, not accepting of their children's emotions, not coaching their children in constructive coping strategies, having marital conflict and domestic violence, and having either neglectful or authoritarian style of parenting (see Chapter 4). Quality of parenting in toddlerhood predicts mental health when the child is an adolescent, so effects occur across time (Kessel et al., 2021).

Are some children just born with a propensity to have emotional disorders? Genes alone are not likely to cause an internalizing disorder, but genes can make some children more vulnerable to the effects of low-quality parenting (Plomin et al., 2016). This means that emotional disorders only develop if children's genetic propensity is combined with low-quality parenting. Ironically, the same genes can make children *less* likely than average to have emotional disorders if they have high-quality parenting.

Psychologists treat emotional disorders in a variety of ways. They can use some of the same approaches discussed in previous chapters to help clients develop better emotion regulation and affective perspective-taking skills. This includes helping clients talk about and label their emotions and helping them learn constructive coping strategies – such as reappraisal, relaxation (for anxiety), and finding an activity that lifts them (for depression). See Box 11.1. Psychologists may also treat emotional disorders by helping clients set realistic goals to develop skills that make the client feel capable. They may point out the progress a client is making. Rather than being critical, psychologists try to create a consistent, responsive, trusting relationship. With young children, psychologists may use play therapy (see Chapter 10).

CBT is a "talk" therapy approach in which psychologists challenge clients' pessimistic thoughts and help them generate more optimistic thoughts. For example, a client may have had a failure experience and feel like a failure in all aspects of life; the therapist helps the client see successes in their life. A client might frame an error at work as a catastrophe that will result in being fired; the therapist helps the client see the error as something small that will not have long-term repercussions. Psychologists may use CBT with people of any age and may combine play therapy with CBT for young children. CBT has been found to be effective for many conditions including depression, anxiety, post-traumatic stress syndrome, panic disorder, fear that one has a serious disease, bulimia, anger control, stress, and others (e.g., Cuijpers et al., 2023; Hofmann et al., 2012). *Trauma-focused CBT* focuses on helping victims process their trauma to develop healthier thought patterns, so they can build resilience and move forward with their lives.

Box 11.1   Interview with a Psychologist

Lisa is a psychologist. She says that psychologists provide a therapeutic relationship for their clients. They also educate their clients and suggest techniques for coping. She helps clients become aware of their own thoughts and emotions and the thoughts and emotions of others. From that awareness, she helps them use coping strategies to handle life's challenges. Psychologists must think about this foundation for healing and emotional growth. Lisa uses this knowledge to teach her clients how to identify and name emotions and how to use appropriate social skills. This leads to competence. Lisa believes that art and music are helpful in work with emotions because they promote reflection, and help clients talk about their emotions. Lisa says that children need to learn social–emotional skills early, such as during transitional kindergarten and elementary school.

Promoting Social Competence

Much of psychologists' work focuses on helping clients improve behavior and have healthy relationships. Common conditions that psychologists deal with in children are oppositional defiant disorder (ODD) and conduct disorder (CD). These are diagnoses given to children who are aggressive, defiant, hostile toward authority figures, annoying to others deliberately, rejecting of blame for their misbehavior, social norm violators, and violators of the rights of others. The diagnoses can range from mild to severe. ODD involves more defiance, and CD involves more aggression. Some children with CD also exhibit callous-unemotional (CU) behavior. This means they hurt others with impunity – their conscience doesn't bother them and they don't respond to others with empathy (Waller et al., 2017). All children misbehave on occasion, but to be diagnosed with ODD or CD, the misbehavior has to be severe enough to disrupt functioning in daily life. Children with these disorders are not likely to have many friends, and their friends are often antisocial.

Just as with internalizing disorders, insecure attachment and low-quality parenting are commonly related to ODD and CD. Compared to securely attached children, insecurely attached children are also more likely to have suicidal thoughts, substance use, eating disorders, poor quality sleep, poor emotion regulation, depression, and anxiety (Al-Yagon & Borenstein, 2022; Dagan et al., 2020; Groh et al., 2017). Their parents are likely to be rejecting, harsh or abusive, drug- and alcohol-using, and have marital conflict. Parents may overreact to their children's behavior with angry, power-assertive discipline which makes it difficult for children to regulate their own emotions. This holds for infants through adolescents. The home life reinforces aggression. Generally, clients with multiple risk factors in their social environment are more likely to develop emotional or behavioral disorders compared with clients with a single risk factor.

Psychologists use CBT to treat externalizing disorders as well as to treat internalizing disorders. This involves helping clients learn problem-solving and conflict resolution skills and learn to think about the consequences of their behavior. It involves *other-oriented induction* such as "how do you think he felt when you ...." CBT helps with managing suicidal ideation. Suicides, although rare, are the second leading cause of death in adolescents and emerging adults.

Psychologists may also use *behavioral therapy*, *applied behavior analysis*, or *functional behavior analysis*, all of which involve applying behaviorism (see Chapter 7) to behavior problems. While these three approaches are not identical, they all involve the following concepts. The psychologist observes what comes before the learner's misbehavior (antecedents) and what consequences (reinforcers) occur after. Reinforcers could include attention from others, escape from teasing, or escape from instruction. The psychologist then changes antecedents and consequences until the misbehavior is reduced. Behavioral psychologists use three principles (Crone et al., 2015):

1. Make the problem behavior unnecessary. If a person is misbehaving to acquire attention, make sure they have adequate attention.
2. Teach a replacement behavior that serves the same function but is more acceptable.
3. Make the problem behavior ineffective for acquiring a reinforcer. However, be warned that eliminating reinforcers can result in increased and stronger attempts to acquire the reinforcer, at least temporarily.

Parenting Training

Psychologists may use family therapy, which involves coaching parents and siblings to be supportive and contribute to the clients' social–emotional progress. For example, family therapy for youth with conduct disorder may focus on parent management training (PMT). This involves training parents, and sometimes *siblings,* to reinforce the target child's prosocial behavior instead of aggression, to use inductive discipline rather than threatening power assertion, to set clear boundaries without being harsh, and to develop good conflict resolution skills. Notice that a key point is to help parents promote prosocial behavior by praising prosocial behavior (see Chapter 2) so that children learn to replace aggression with kindness. Psychologists may also use parent–child interaction therapy (PCIT) which involves coaching parents *while* they are interacting their child. When working with parents, psychologists may need to support them through frustration, anger, and exhaustion if they are trying to care for a child with mental or behavioral problems.

Repairing Attachment

As you come to understand the importance of secure attachment, you can see why therapy often centers on supporting clients in overcoming a history of insecure attachment. Because we tend to parent in the same way we were parented, security of attachment is transmitted across generations. So how can psychologists disrupt insecure attachment across generations? Psychologists seek to build trust and emotional security in parent–child relationships in order to repair attachment. The purpose of attachment-based therapy (ABT) is to help parents become more sensitive and responsive to their child's emotional needs and learn to interpret the child's behavior accurately. For example, one mother in therapy believed that her infant was "just trying to manipulate" her because he would fuss if left in the highchair with nothing to do for long periods of time. The psychologist worked with her to see the infants' perspective and re-interpret his behavior as normal infant behavior. The infant needed to be free to move, he needed a toy or something to explore, and he needed someone to talk to and smile at him. Fortunately, research has found that when parents are trained to be more sensitive, their children's attachment security improves. With older youth and emerging adults, psychologists help clients explore how their early childhood experiences of attachment are affecting current relationships and feelings. Fortunately, research has found that when parents are trained to be more sensitive, their children's attachment security improves (see Figure 11.1).

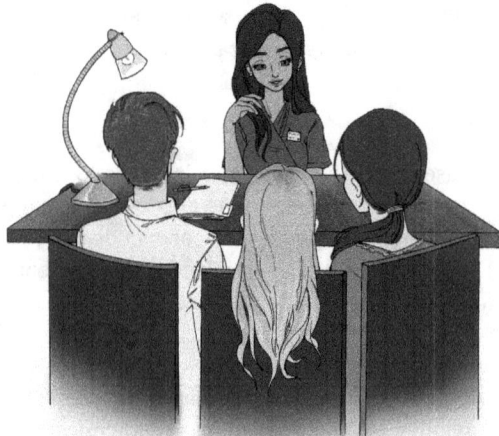

Figure 11.1 Therapy that focuses on parenting helps many families address mental and behavioral challenges in youth.

Relationship Therapy

Psychologists may use interpersonal therapy (IPT) that focuses on improving relationships. For example, psychologists may help the client navigate interpersonal issues, such as conflict resolution skills. Psychologists may help clients examine whether their relationships are healthy. They may teach clients the ABCs of healthy relationships: Awareness (i.e., see clearly what is happening in family, friend, or romantic relationships), Balance (i.e., there is balance in the relationship with give and take, but no one dominates or controls the other), and Creativity (i.e., each feels free to learn and grow and support each other through changes). Unhealthy relationships are controlling, hostile, destructive, dishonest, or even violent. The psychologist might ask questions like "Do you feel like you can tell the truth to each other? Can you talk openly about feelings, even when it is hard? Do you treat each other with respect? Do you both compromise sometimes?" Some clients need to learn that in healthy family relationships or friendships there is some conflict, but these are "good" disagreements where participants are able to work through conflict. In healthy relationships, one feels safe, responsibilities and boundaries are clear, and each has the other's best interest at heart. In a two-person relationship, both should be sincere, honest, supportive, and prosocial. Psychologists try to model this when working with emerging adults by building rapport, being compassionate, actively listening (rather than being judgmental), being respectful, empowering the client by allowing them to choose therapy options, and validating their emotions and experiences.

Chapter Summary

While research psychologists do research that may or may not have direct implications for helping people, applied psychologists work directly with children and adults to improve their well-being. Applied psychologists may work in schools, hospitals, or private offices. This chapter focuses on applied psychologists. Different types of applied psychologists require different types and levels of training.

Insecure attachment is a primary cause of internalizing and externalizing disorders. This is why therapy often centers on supporting clients in overcoming a history of insecure attachment, fostering more sensitive parenting, and helping clients learn to have healthy social relationships. Different approaches to therapy (e.g., play or art therapy, CBT, PMT, PCIT, IPT, ABT) have been found to be effective in promoting clients' social–emotional competencies.

References

Al-Yagon, M., & Borenstein, T. (2022). Adolescents' executive functions: Links to inattention, hyperactivity-impulsivity, trait mindfulness, and attachment relationships with fathers and mothers. *Research in Developmental Disabilities, 124*, 104212.

Crone, D. A., Hawken, L. S., & Horner, R. H. (2015). *Building positive behavior support systems in schools: Functional behavioral assessment* (2nd ed.). Guilford.

Cuijpers, P., Miguel, C., Harrer, M., Plessen, C.Y., Ciharova, M., Ebert, D., & Karyotaki, E. (2023). Cognitive behavior therapy vs. control conditions, other psychotherapies, pharmacotherapies and combined treatment for depression: A comprehensive meta-analysis including 409 trials with 52,702 patients. *World Psychiatry, 22*(1), 105–115.

Dagan, O., Facompré, C. R., Nivison, M. D., Roisman, G. I., & Bernard, K. (2020). Preoccupied and dismissing attachment representations are differentially associated with anxiety in adolescence and adulthood: A meta-analysis. *Clinical Psychological Science, 8*(4), 614–640.

Deneault, A.-A., Bakermans-Kranenburg, M. J., Groh, A. M., Fearon, P. R. M., &Madigan, S. (2021). Child-father attachment in early childhood and behavior problems: A meta-analysis. *New Directions for Child and Adolescent Development, 2021*, 43–66.

Groh, A. M., Fearon, R. M. P., van Ijzendoorn, M. H., Bakermans-Kranenburg, M. J., & Roisman, G. I. (2017). Attachment in the early life course: Meta-analytic evidence for its role in socioemotional development. *Child Development Perspectives, 11*(1), 70–76.

Gross, J. J., & Jazaieri, H. (2014). Emotion, emotion regulation, and psychopathology: An affective science perspective. *Clinical Psychological Science, 2*(4), 387–401.

Hofmann, S.G., Asnaani, A., Vonk, I., Sawyer, A., & Fang, A. (2012). The efficacy of cognitive behavioral therapy: A review of meta-analyses. *Cognitive Therapy and Research, 36*, 427–440.

Kessel, E. M., Dougherty, L. R., Hubacheck, S., Chad-Friedman, E., Olino, T., Carlson, G. A., & Klein, D. N. (2021). Early predictors of adolescent irritability. *Child and Adolescent Psychiatric Clinics of North America, 30*(3), 475–490.

Krokstad S, Weiss D., Krokstad M., Rangul, V., Kvaløy, K., Ingul, M., Bjerkeset, O., Twenge, J., & Sund, E. (2022). Divergent decennial trends in mental health according to age reveal poorer mental health for young people: Repeated cross-sectional population-based surveys from the HUNT Study, Norway. *BMJ Open, 12*, e057654.

Parodi, K.B., Holt, M.K., Green, J.G., Porche, M., Koenig, B., & Ziming, X. (2022). Time trends and disparities in anxiety among adolescents, 2012–2018. *Social Psychiatry and Psychiatric Epidemiology, 57*, 127–137.

Plomin, R., DeFries, J. C., Knopik, V. S., & Neiderhiser, J. M. (2016). Top 10 replicated findings from behavioral genetics. *Perspectives on Psychological Science, 11*(1), 3–23.

Santomauro, D. and COVID-19 Mental Disorders Collaborators. (2021). Global prevalence and burden of depressive and anxiety disorders in 204 countries and territories in 2020 due to the COVID-19 pandemic. *The Lancet, 398*(10312), 1700–1712.

Waller, R., Shaw, D. S., & Hyde, L. W. (2017). Observed fearlessness and positive parenting interact to predict childhood callous-unemotional behaviors among low-income boys. *Journal of Child Psychology and Psychiatry, and Allied Disciplines, 58*(3), 282–291.

Index

For Product Safety Concerns and Information please contact our EU
representative GPSR@taylorandfrancis.com
Taylor & Francis Verlag GmbH, Kaufingerstraße 24, 80331 München, Germany

www.ingramcontent.com/pod-product-compliance
Lightning Source LLC
Chambersburg PA
CBHW070341270326
41926CB00017B/3933